the live-long code

€7.99

Also by Dermot O'Connor

The Healing Code

the live-long code

dermot o'connor

unlocking the secrets to a longer,
healthier and happier life

HACHETTE
BOOKS
IRELAND

To my children, Faye, Alison and Grace.

This is for you in the hope that your dad and your fantastic mom,
Fiona, will be here for you for a very, very long time.

To Yvonne, without your love and support
this book would never have happened.

And to Aunt Helen, thank you for everything.

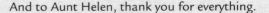

First published in Ireland in 2009 by Hachette Books Ireland
First published in paperback in 2010 by Hachette Books Ireland
A Hachette UK company

1

Copyright © Dermot O'Connor 2009

The right of Dermot O'Connor to be identified as the Author of the Work has
been asserted by him in accordance with the Copyright, Designs and Patents Act 1988.

The information contained in this book has been obtained from reliable sources.
However it is intended as a guideline only and should never be used as a replacement
for consultation with your regular physician. While every effort has been made to
ensure accuracy no responsibility for loss, damage or injury occassioned to any
person acting or refraining from action as a result of information contained herein
can be accepted by the publishers or author.

Photography by Agata Stoinska

A CIP catalogue record for this title is available from the British Library.

ISBN 978 0 340 95089 0

Typeset in Legacy Serif Book by Hewer Text UK Ltd, Edinburgh
Printed and bound by CPI Mackays, Chatham ME5 8TD

Hachette Books Ireland policy is to use papers that are natural, renewable and
recyclable products and made from wood grown in sustainable forests. The
logging and manufacturing processes are expected to conform to the
environmental regulations of the country of origin.

Hachette Books Ireland
8 Castlecourt Centre
Castleknock
Dublin 15

www.hachette.ie

Contents

The Live-Long Code is also known as The Immortality Code. More details can be found on www.immortalitycode.com

Foreword

Living life to the full involves some simple things. Health. Love. Harmony with the world around us. A productive life of honest achievement, friendship and fun with our fellow man.

Anyone who has read Dermot's previous book, *The Healing Code*, knows the importance of all these blessings. *The Healing Code* has pride of place on my own bookshelf, and it contains many words of wisdom and sound guidance for regaining and retaining the vitality we need to enjoy our time on this earth.

But how much time do we really have? Conventional wisdom allots us our three-score years and ten, before we must take our leave of this world and say goodbye to those we love.

But what if conventional wisdom is wrong? What if there is a way to hold on to this cherished life of ours, and all its bounteous gifts, for extra years, decades even? What if we could sweep aside the boundaries to our enjoyment of life, and face the prospect of limitless time, limitless health?

In the past, these questions have been mere riddles, thought experiments to help us understand how positive we feel about our lives, or whether we have become tired of the toil and responsibility that comes with life and experience. Would we choose our lives time after time, or would we willingly shuffle off our mortal coils and choose an oblivion of endless rest and peace?

For my part, life itself has always been the ultimate joy, and there comes no greater peace or satisfaction than facing up to the challenges life brings, overcoming them, conquering them. Give me the challenges, the hardships, triumphs and occasional failures of life over the uneventful peace of eternity. I embrace all these facets of life with my mantra: "Every day you can get out of bed is a great day."

If you are like me, if you want to make life better, more vibrant, more healthy and more limitless, then this book is for you.

My own life has been one of overcoming limits. There are the limits that other people, or society, seeks to place upon us from childhood. The limits that our rivals and competitors place in our path, that we must overcome to succeed in life, in business and in love. And, most pernicious of all, there are the limits we can set upon ourselves, the limits of what we hope for and what we dare to believe.

I believe that limits are there to be extended, and my life bears testament to this. Although I was expelled from school at the age of thirteen, I was appointed managing director of a large car dealership with a staff of one hundred at the age of twenty-two. I went on to become one of the first Irishmen to achieve a multinational car distribution franchise. I was the first Irishman to walk the Channel Tunnel from France to England. I have been fortunate enough to pen the biggest-selling Irish biography in history, *A Long Way from Penny Apples*. Soon, I will be the first Irishman to journey into space and, at the age of sixty-seven, I am still "pushing the envelope". I do not expect that enthusiasm and focus to end any time soon.

That is why I am so delighted with Dermot's new book *The Live-Long Code*. Its very title is a challenge to us to believe something new, to set aside the limits and conventions that keep us from believing the impossible. It reminds me of what my grandmother Moll Darcy said to me many times. "Take responsibility for your health, son, and respect the wonders God gave you." She lived to be one hundred.

Dermot's approach is one that we can all believe in. He takes the very latest in cutting-edge health science, allies it to age-old wisdom from the ancient masters of Chinese traditional medicine, and completes the mix with a healthy optimism based on the coming advances in medical technology, which we are only now beginning to experience. His conclusion? The limits of health-span and lifespan, the surly bonds of earth and time, are weakening now, stretching out, and the horizon of life and happiness is expanding faster and faster. For those of us with ears to listen, Dermot tells us exactly what we should be doing – the foods and nourishment we should take to sustain our bodies, and the behaviour and attitudes we should cultivate to sustain our souls and our minds – to give ourselves every chance of reaping the benefits of the new age that stretches before us.

Dermot's new book is a tonic for the soul and body. I have always believed that, whether or not our lives have an unknown and unknowable boundary, we should live as though eternity stretched before us. With *The Live-Long Code,* I am more convinced than ever that what I have always known, instinctively, might – just might – turn out to be true after all.

Several years ago, I booked my one hundredth birthday party for Dromoland Castle. It's still a long way away, but today, having read Dermot's marvellous book, I'm thinking of booking my two hundredth as well. Why don't *you* come on this wonderful journey with me and Dermot O'Connor.

Bill Cullen
Host of *The Apprentice* Irish TV series
Author of *Its a Long Way From Penny Apples* and
Golden Apples: Six Simple Steps to Success

Introduction

The human body is designed for longevity. This is demonstrated by the many hundreds of thousands of long-lived and healthy people around the world. Our bodies are genetically 'programmed' to live beyond the hundred years that many of us still see as exceptional.

The belief that ageing is an inescapable process that involves the rapid degradation of the mind and body is considered the acceptable norm. We all want to grow old slowly, but we know little about how to grow old healthily. We continually subject our bodies to all kinds of physical, mental and emotional abuse, as if we were somehow separate from our bodies. We think of our bodies as vehicles that have nothing to do with us; provided they are not inconvenienced by illness or injury, we are shocked when the machinery stops working correctly – and ultimately shuts down completely.

In a way, our bodies *can* be compared to an everyday piece of machinery such as a car. If you take care of your car – providing it with the right fuel and oil, polishing and cleaning it inside and out, taking it to the garage frequently to get it serviced – it will go on and on, providing many years of satisfactory driving. However, if you neglect your car – ignoring service checks, not checking tyres, not changing the oil or, worse still, using the wrong type of fuel – it won't be long before it lets you down, possibly permanently.

Of course we are infinitely more complex than a car or any man-made mechanism. In fact, part of our complexity is our inbuilt capacity to repair ourselves. We human beings consist of mind, body and spirit and there are strong links between the exchanges of energy and biological mutations that make us live. These intimate connections give us the perception of being alive, and continuously stabilise and renew the life force within us. The ageing process can be seen as the build-up of defects that disturb the normal processes of life. It takes ill health, or the loss of good health, to take us off the road.

This quest for immortality has a long tradition in both Eastern and Western medical and scientific cultures. Modern biochemistry has its roots in the world of alchemy, where notable scientists such as Isaac Newton and Robert Boyle showed a keen interest in the search for the Philosopher's Stone – the substance that would transform base metals into gold, which was believed to carry life-extending powers and act as a universal panacea. Similarly, many of the great historical masters of Chinese medicine devoted much of their effort to the pursuit of the Grand Elixir of Immortality.

While this age-old quest hasn't yet yielded immortality, the latest scientific research indicates that a life expectancy in excess of 100 years should be achievable for most of us. We can remain in good working order, in full possession of our physical and mental capacities, for at least a century – and in principle, for considerably longer, as shown by the table below.

Life Expectancy

Neanderthal – 30,000 BC	20 years
Palaeolithic – 10,000 BC	33 years
Bronze Age – 2,000 BC	18 years
Classical Greek – 300 BC	25 years
Classical Roman – AD 500	25 years
Medieval Britain – AD 1300	25 years
Early 20th century	35 years
Current world average	78 years
Predicted world average in AD 2050	90 years*
Predicted world average in AD 2100	5,000 years**

*Source: University of Southern California
** Source: Aubrey de Grey, longevity scientist, Cambridge University

Although you might consider aiming for an average lifespan of 100 years to be an unrealistic goal, if you look at average life expectancy through history, you can see that we have already made very considerable strides towards this. At the turn of the twentieth century, average life expectancy was less than half what it is now and had been approximately the same for thousands of years. We have therefore dramatically increased life expectancy in the past 100 years, and it is reasonable to postulate that this trend will continue. Indeed, prominent scientists such as Aubrey de Grey now consider it possible that we are on the verge of seeing the average human lifespan reach 200 years, or even more. This might seem farfetched, but consider other advances in biotechnology that have made possible events such as the 67-year-old Spanish woman who in 2006 became the world's oldest mother after she gave birth to twins in Barcelona.

We will touch on the area of cutting-edge longevity research later in the book, but for the moment we can use the knowledge already in our possession to maximise our potential to extend our healthy lives. Progress towards an average lifespan of 100 years or more is now attainable through an improvement in lifestyle, a more in-depth knowledge of the body and what suits it best and listening carefully to what our bodies are telling us.

Over the past few decades we have seen the development of medical knowledge around disorders associated with the ageing process. As we understand it now, the central issue in increasing lifespan is identifying the techniques for heading off the ageing process. In other words, the principles of healthier living have become the main focus of longevity research. *The Live-Long Code* identifies the key emerging breakthroughs in the different strands of health and longevity research, and brings them together in a way that will extend your lifespan – and equally importantly, your health span – to the edges of human possibility.

The Elements of the Live-Long Code

What is science telling us about how to extend our period of life and health? These are the elements of the Live-Long Code that will be outlined in this book.

- We start from the principle of listening to our body rather than trying to conquer it or make it subject to our will. Our bodies are not separate from ourselves – we *are* our bodies, and our first duty is to allow our body's own health-giving processes to function freely.
- Modern nutritional science has produced a comparatively robust and well-understood set of principles for eating healthily. Identifying these principles and putting them into practice is a cornerstone of the Live-Long Code.
- Similarly, performing the optimal kind and amount of exercise for prolonging health, maintaining mental agility and making a conscious contribution to the functioning of our circulation, breathing, digestion and mental health will all play a part in allowing us to successfully add many healthy and happy years to our lives.

Taken as a whole, the Live-Long Code approach creates a direct involvement in and responsibility for the life of our body. By taking good care of ourselves every day, we can retain the harmony of mind and body. By learning about longevity and the prevention or slowing down of ageing, we listen to ourselves more. The illnesses and diseases that become more prevalent with age should not be thought of as an inevitable part of the human condition, but rather as accidents that are possible to avoid or prevent – just as, when driving a car along the motorway, we can navigate carefully to avoid the hazards that come our way, and so continue peacefully on our journey.

As someone who has helped thousands of people combat illness, I am committed to this battle against the diseases of ageing. How can we live better and longer and make full use of our genetic code? A clear analysis of ourselves and our bodies will enable us to understand how the ageing process really occurs and how it can be forestalled.

It is usually when things go wrong that we start to notice that we are growing old. It is from this moment, or even better, from before this moment arrives, that it is important to take remedial action, to take charge of and responsibility for ourselves. Maximising our body's ability to renew itself involves a partnership between modern medicine, with all its advances and discoveries, and the wisdom of centuries, together with your own willingness to know yourself and to work on avoiding the dangers of old age. Nothing can be established if your doctor doesn't take your biological strengths and weaknesses into consideration, but first of all you need to know yourself. The code to healthy long living requires a good understanding of yourself so that you can identify your health risk factors, understand the mechanisms of your body and take a complete look at your lifestyle. The Live-Long Code is a radical plan for life extension, an evolving plan which involves the evaluation of various health-risk factors. The plan set out in this book provides vital information, based on the latest cutting-edge advances in science, for:

- assessing your total health profile;
- assessing your cellular ageing profile and the deterioration of the cellular membranes;
- understanding the psychology and mental approach to healthy longer living;
- implementing the optimal nutritional plan for longevity; and
- creating the best exercise approach to healthy life extension.

Through the ages, for most people the secrets of ageing well or badly have seemed to lie in unknown forces such as DNA, God and fate. Whatever one's faith, for centuries there seemed to be no concrete reason why one person would outlive another. Why one person would suffer the ravages of time more than another. Why illness and early death would come to one person's door and not another's. For many years people have tended to believe that they could not effectively influence how long they would live or the quality of life they would have as they aged.

Recent scientific discoveries have, however, revealed some startling new insights into our biological make-up. We now understand that we humans can take strong action to slow down the ageing process and gain significant influence over our health as we age. Scientific discoveries will soon develop further, into new technologies that will increase the distance between an individual's actual calendar age and their biological age, or the condition and health of their body.

Of course living longer in itself makes no real sense unless you are healthy enough to enjoy those extra years and decades. And this is exactly the aim of the Live-Long Code – to help you to live longer and prolong youthfulness and vitality into your later years. The tools necessary to achieve this lie for the most part within you.

The secret of the Live-Long Code anti-ageing programme lies in the details – details tailored to your body and your needs. It is through understanding and applying the principles of the Live-Long Code Programme that you will be able to access and follow a complete, thorough and successful personal anti-ageing programme.

For *The Live-Long Code,* I have examined the growing field of anti-ageing medicine. I have cut through the conflicting information to reveal what you can do right now and what treatments may be available in the future to help you on your way.

We have established that positive lifestyle choices result in longer living. When we look at the longest-lived people in the world we notice that while the ageing process continues, the incidence of age-related diseases – cancer, heart disease, Alzheimer's – drops. It is almost as if there is a switch in the body that reacts to this natural ageing situation. As if, internally, there is a realisation that if you can get this far along healthily, you should continue along the path of good health.

My aim in this book is to help you achieve what thousands of my clients have experienced by reaching their optimum health goals. I want to get you to the point where you are healthy and ready to live longer, free of disease and of sound mind. So let's begin our journey.

CHAPTER ONE
What Is Ageing?

Ageing has always been thought of as the inevitable consequence of time. We accept that the longer we live, the more our bodies and minds will deteriorate. Just as a car erodes slowly over time, becoming more and more unreliable until one day it stops working altogether, so time takes its inevitable toll on our bodies, which become more decrepit as we age. If the biological clock continues for long enough, so traditional thinking goes, our deterioration is inevitable. Or so we thought until recently. As scientists continue to probe and investigate the ageing process, the old preconceptions of what constitutes ageing are being profoundly challenged.

In the brave new world of anti-ageing medicine, ageing itself is considered by many to be a disease. As such, the thinking is that through proper intervention it can be prevented, or at least postponed. The cumulative effect of diseases caused by a lifetime's exposure to environmental and lifestyle assault is a slow breakdown of the body, culminating in the deterioration of bodily functions – what is termed 'chronic disease'. To use the analogy of the car, the scratches and dents on the body do not occur naturally, but appear over time as the inevitable consequence of careless collisions and reckless driving.

Illnesses such as osteoporosis, heart disease, stroke, cancer, arthritis, Parkinson's disease and multiple sclerosis, to name just a few, generally have ageing and cellular deterioration as their common components. These afflictions most frequently occur after the age of 40, which is generally considered to be a pivot point between youth and old age. In addition to this, many medical scientists now believe that structures within the human genetic code moderate the pace of ageing, and furthermore that these genetic structures

7

can be modified. The use of antioxidants to prevent and even treat serious conditions such as heart disease, cancer and arthritis indicates that ageing can itself be thought of as a disease. Why? Because as noted, these conditions correlate closely with the ageing process itself.

Just as the metal body of a car is prone to rusting – or oxidation, to give the process its chemical name – so too are our bodies subject to attack from natural oxidative processes. Oxidation or the 'rusting' of our body actually begins very early in life; it does not occur only in old age. Oxidation can be thought of as an external assault on our natural life processes, whereby free radical damage essentially leads to ageing and the chronic diseases of old age.

How Can We Treat Ageing?

When we accept the proposition that ageing is itself a disease, it becomes easier to accept that ageing is both treatable and preventable. Scientific studies of the genetic code of DNA in chronic illnesses such as cancer, cardiovascular disease and neurological disorders suggest that oxidation plays a major role in their development.

However, it is now understood that much of this deterioration can be amended by eating food rich in antioxidants. Furthermore, it has been found that antioxidant supplements can contribute to replenishing cells harmed by oxidation.

Hopefully this will help you see that, armed with the right information, you can direct yourself towards a long life of good health and well being. The first step of this journey is to acquire information, so we will spend some time looking at the theories of ageing. The details and practices disclosed in this book derive from the knowledge that is at the heart of the most up-to-date anti-ageing medicine and illness prevention. By following this step-by-step programme, you will set yourself on the journey to continued good health and you will be able to buy time to take advantage of the amazing medical and anti-ageing discoveries that are just around the corner. Prominent scientists postulate that with these imminent breakthroughs it may be possible for people who are already as old as 60 to live to be 150. Knowledge of the Live-Long Code can also increase your prospects of surviving the vulnerable period of your seventies and eighties, helping you to increase your chances of avoiding Alzheimer's disease, stroke, heart attack and other potentially devastating illnesses.

However, knowledge alone is not enough and it is only through continuous and concerted commitment to practising the Live-Long Code that your endeavour will be rewarded. Extending one's life in order to get the most out of it takes dedication. With this programme in your arsenal, you will have the weapons to fight a heroic battle against encroaching age.

Why the Growth of Anti-Ageing Medicine?

Anti-ageing medicine is a fast-growing industry. Why? Well, centenarians are the fastest-growing demographic group in most developed countries. In 1963 there were only 153 centenarians in the whole of Japan. By 2006 this number had grown to 28,395. By the year 2050, the average lifespan may well reach 90 years and the number of centenarians will be in the millions.

For many, the prospect of growing older is not necessarily a pleasant one to ponder, as most people associate this time of life with decrepitude. However, this will all change. As advanced anti-ageing medicines develop, these later years will not be marred by incapacity and frailty, but by productivity and robustness. This will be the dawn of literally a new age for older people, when in effect they will be younger than their calendar years indicate.

Let's now look at the symptoms of ageing in order to get a clearer picture of what it really entails.

How We Age

Most people would probably say that ageing begins in our thirties, when wrinkles start to appear and hair begins to lose volume and perhaps change colour. Physical ailments may also start to appear more frequently. However, a closer look at a microbiological level reveals that the symptoms of ageing often begin long before our thirties.

The Brain – Ageing Starts at 20

As we age the number of cells, or neurons, in our brain decreases. We start with around 100 billion, but by our twenties this has started to decline and by our late thirties we are losing 10,000 neurons a day. Although neuroscientists calculate that we have billions upon billions of neurons to spare, this chronic decay can affect many aspects of our brain's functioning, including co-ordination, memory and even language skills. However, while these neurons are important, it is the deterioration of the gaps between the brain cells that carries the greatest impact. These tiny gaps are called synapses and their job is to facilitate the flow of information from one cell to another. It is important to mention that the process of synaptic decay can be arrested and even reversed through mental exercise techniques.

The Lungs – Ageing Starts at 20

Lung capacity starts to decline from as early as 20. By the age of 40 many people are already experiencing breathlessness. The muscles of the ribcage can stiffen as we get older and hinder our breathing. This then makes it harder for the lungs to work, and also means that some air remains in the lungs after breathing out, which causes breathlessness. An average man of 30 can inhale a litre of air in one breath, but by the age of 70 this capacity has decreased to just half of that amount.

More effort is then required to move air in and out of the lungs, and more air is retained in the lungs after exhaling. The amount of oxygen-to-blood transfer also decreases with age. Consequently, with less air and less oxygen in the bloodstream there is a decrease in the amount of work that can be performed. More far-reaching consequences may also occur if there is a significant decrease in the amount of oxygen reaching the brain; symptoms like disorientation, confusion, memory loss and insomnia are all quite common.

The Skin – Ageing Starts Mid-Twenties

The skin starts to age in our mid-twenties. As we get older the production of collagen, the protein that acts like scaffolding for the skin, decreases. Elastin, the substance that enables the skin to snap back into place, loses its spring as the skin ages and can even break. Dead skin cells don't shed as quickly as we age and the production of new skin cells also decreases. This causes fine lines and wrinkles to form and the first outward signs of ageing to appear. This is accelerated by factors such as sun damage and smoking.

The Muscles – Ageing Starts at 30

Muscles are constantly built up and broken down. This process is well balanced in young, healthy adults, but usually by the age of 30 the breakdown is faster than the build-up. By the time we reach 40 the average person is losing up to 2 per cent of their muscle each year.

The Hair – Ageing Starts at 30

Hair loss usually begins in our thirties, although genetic factors can accelerate or delay this process. Hair is made from tiny pockets under the skin's surface called follicles. A hair normally grows from each follicle for about three years, is shed and then a new hair grows. However, changes in testosterone levels can affect this cycle and cause the hair follicle to shrink. This results in the new hairs becoming increasingly thinner until all that remains is a much smaller hair follicle and then a stump of hair that doesn't grow beyond the skin's surface. Most people will have some grey hair by the age of 35. When we are younger our hair colour is produced and maintained by pigments in the hair follicle called melanocytes. However, as we age these melanocytes become less active and produce less pigment. The colour fades and the absence of colour has a greying effect on the hair.

The Bones – Ageing Starts at 35

Old bone is broken down by cells called osteoclasts and is replaced by bone-building cells called osteoblasts. This process is called bone turnover and decelerates rapidly as we get older. A child's skeleton renews itself completely in just 2 years, but the process slows and can take up to 10 years in an adult.

Until our mid-twenties, our bone density is constantly increasing, but by our mid-thirties bone-density loss begins. It accelerates further in post-menopausal women and can cause the bone-thinning condition osteoporosis. This shrinking in the size and density of bones is responsible for the loss of height that frequently comes with ageing, as the bones in the back shrivel or crumble. By the age of 80 the average person has lost 2 inches in height.

Fertility – Ageing Starts at 35

Female fertility begins to decline after 35 as the quantity and quality of eggs produced in the ovaries starts to decline. The lining of the womb may also become thinner, making it less likely for a fertilised egg to take and making the environment harder for sperm to survive in. Although male fertility lasts longer, the quality of sperm produced by a man after the age of 40 is generally poorer as he ages.

The Eyes – Ageing Starts at 40

Most people have failing eyesight by the time they reach their forties. This usually comes in the form of long-sightedness, which affects our ability to see close-up objects. This is because our eye muscles become weaker with age and so our ability to focus deteriorates. At around 50 the ability to see clearly at night decreases, and the ability to see fine detail declines around the age of 70. The possibility of macular degeneration (the progressive deterioration of the retina) rises sharply after the age of about 60.

The Teeth – Ageing Starts at 40

As we age we produce less saliva. Saliva's function is to wash away bacteria and help protect the teeth and gums. Receding gums, when tissue is lost from around the teeth because they are not adequately protected, is common in most adults over about 40.

The Heart – Ageing Starts at 40
The heart's ability to pump blood decreases as we get older. This is due to blood vessels losing their elasticity, while arteries can also harden or become more blocked due to fatty deposits forming on the coronary arteries. The blood supply to the heart is therefore reduced and can result in angina. Men over 45 and women over 55 are therefore at greater risk of heart attack. Recent research has found that the average person's heart age is five years older than their actual age due to obesity and a lack of exercise.

The Prostate – Ageing Starts at 50
The prostate gland often becomes enlarged with age, leading to issues such as a need to urinate with increased frequency and urgency. This condition is known as benign prostatic hyperplasia and it affects half the men over 50. It occurs when the prostate starts absorbing large amounts of the male sex hormone testosterone, which then causes an increase in the growth of cells in the prostate.

Hearing – Ageing Starts Mid-Fifties
More than 50 per cent of people over the age of 60 start to lose their hearing. This condition, known as presbycusis, is due to the loss of the tiny sensory cells in the inner ear known as hair cells, which pick up sound vibrations and send them to the brain.

Kidneys – Ageing Starts at 50
The number of filtering units, or nephrons, in the kidneys starts to decline in our fifties. Nephrons remove waste from the bloodstream, and one result of their decline is an inability to switch off urine production at night – which results in frequent visits to the bathroom at night-time. The kidneys of a 75-year-old filter only half the amount of blood as those of a 30-year-old.

The Gut – Ageing Starts at 55

The gastrointestinal tract, or gut, is our system of digestive organs. A healthy gut maintains a good balance between harmful and friendly bacteria, but the levels of friendly bacteria in the gut drop significantly after the age of 55 and as a result we can start to suffer from poor digestion and increased risk of gut disease. Constipation is also more common as we age, as the flow of digestive juices from the stomach, liver, pancreas and small intestine starts to slow down.

The Bladder – Ageing Starts at 65

Loss of bladder control becomes far more common after 65. Women are more vulnerable to bladder difficulties than men, as declining oestrogen levels make the tissues of the urethra – the tube through which urine passes – thinner and weaker, reducing bladder support.

The bladder capacity in an older adult is usually about half the amount of that of a young adult, which means more frequent and urgent trips to the loo as we age. Poor muscle tone around the bladder can lessen the ability to empty the bladder fully and can result in urinary tract infections.

The Liver – Ageing Starts at 70

This is the only organ in the body that seems to defy the ageing process; its cells show an extraordinary capacity to regenerate. Half a liver can be removed and within just three months it will grow back to the size of a complete liver.

It is easy to see why the march toward old age is often pejoratively referred to as 'the steady slide downward'. Yet it seems almost ironic, or perhaps tragic, that just when many people begin to live in the fullness of life, degeneration of all sorts strikes them. It is equally easy to understand why many people feel cheated. From this standpoint, it seems only fair that the prime of life should be extended and spent in good health – that is, through at least the sixth, seventh, eighth and ninth decades of life.

Can We Increase Lifespan?

There has probably never been a period in human history in which lifespan has not been increasing, with a few exceptions such as during the plagues of the Middle Ages. Generally speaking, human lifespan has been slowly but steadily increasing.

Over a period of almost 1,500 years, human lifespan only increased by four years. Within the past century, though, it has nearly doubled. This is mainly due to increased awareness of the importance of hygiene and sanitation and the dramatic drop in infant mortality. As we move into the twenty-first century, many in the scientific community believe that we are poised to make other important gains in life extension.

Many ongoing studies are starting to report dramatic increases in animal lifespan in experimental environments. One such study has shown that rats that have their food intake cut by 40 per cent have lived as much as 70 per cent longer. Also, interestingly, they are largely free of diabetes, cancer and heart disease. When they do get these diseases, they get them much later compared to animals that eat all they want. These calorie-restriction studies have now been extended to include other species, including primates, and are showing similar results.

Human studies are now under way and scientists expect them to yield similar results. The studies of the Okinawans of Japan indicate that one of the reasons why they are the longest-living people on the planet is their tendency to eat less food than the rest of us.

Another interesting experiment was the Biosphere Project. From 1991 to 1993, eight men and women were locked away from the world in a sealed, self-contained artificial dome and tasked with growing their own food, maintaining their own air supply and recycling all their water within the closed ecosystem. When the group ran low on food, something interesting happened. As the team members ate less, their body statistics changed. The men lost an average of 18 per cent body weight, the women 10 per cent. Blood pressure fell by an average of 20 per cent. Indicators for diabetes, such as blood sugar and insulin levels, decreased by 30 per cent on average and cholesterol levels also dropped. In other words, as the group ate less, the biomarkers of health indicated that they were healthier.

In another experiment, conducted by geneticist Dr Cynthia Kenyon, when the daf-2 gene in worms was altered the worms lived for a month on average, doubling the previous average of two weeks. It was also noted that these genetically modified worms not only lived longer but also lived more healthily. In a parallel study of other genetically altered worms, researchers established that these worms ate less, defecated less and lived longer – in fact, they lived for the human equivalent of 375 years.

The possibilities for further breakthroughs in lifespan increase are very promising. In the past generation the average lifespan has increased more dramatically than in any other time in human history, so with new drugs and new experiments in genetics and other ventures, we can reasonably expect even further increases.

Why Do We Age?

There are many theories about the causes of ageing, but it is most likely that ageing is a result of a combination of the factors in these theories. Experts agree that maintaining wellness into advanced age is the key to promoting longevity and preventing disease. The Live-Long Code defines successful ageing as the ability to live a happy, healthy and productive life into the tenth decade and even beyond. Increasing longevity involves many components, including genetics, but health is not dependent on genes alone and no matter what genes you have, following a healthy lifestyle like the one laid out in the Live-Long Code is the most critical factor.

Evolutionary biologist George C. Williams found that lifestyle and environmental factors have a direct effect on our genetic code. So while genetics may programme ageing up to a point, they are influenced by environmental and lifestyle factors as well, inter-acting with one another to determine our personal ageing process. Since lifestyle plays such a crucial role, you have the power to control your longevity through diet, mental approach, nutritional supplements, exercise and the avoidance of toxins. *The Live-Long Code* contains the most up-to-date knowledge on how to incorporate longevity techniques into your life and presents a comprehensive approach to modifying your lifestyle factors as well as promoting positive genetic expression and minimising negative genetic tendencies.

To withstand the causes of ageing you need a consistent and sustained approach to prolonging your health. You also need to develop the correct mental approach and philosophy of life to deal with the rigours of living.

As you read *The Live-Long Code* you will become aware that healthy ageing is enhanced by lifelong good health, and that although you can implement the Live-Long Code at any age, the sooner you start, the better. At the core of this book is a belief that a lifestyle that promotes optimal health, supported by natural medicine and practised continuously throughout a lifetime, will foster greatly enhanced longevity.

But before we detail the strategic approach of the Live-Long Code, let's look at what scientists are saying about ageing and examine the importance of the way we look at ageing and how we live as we age. Armed with this information, you will understand the principles and will be able to implement the Live-Long Code more effectively and efficiently.

The Study of Ageing

To fully understand ageing we need to look at the process from many points of view – chemical, biological and psychological. We must take account of the latest and most advanced knowledge that medical science can provide. But it would be sensible to also include the ancient and time-proven knowledge of Eastern sciences and arts. Chinese medical scholars have not only extensively studied the effects of ageing, but have also developed and practised longevity techniques and developed pragmatic approaches to extending lifespan. In fact, although most of us probably think of anti-ageing medicine as a modern phenomenon, the search for immortality and revealing how to prolong life have always been seen as the holy grail of Chinese medicine, with many of its most prominent practitioners throughout history devoting much of their lives to the search for this noble treasure.

The study of ageing can be difficult for a variety of reasons. One reason is that it occurs slowly and – hopefully – over a long period of time. Another reason is that, particularly in the past, there were few people who lived long enough to provide a proper study group. However, there are individuals who have already navigated the journey to 100 years and older, and by studying them we can glean clues about successful ageing. The most well-known study of this kind is the Okinawa Centenarian Study, a 25-year study of the longest-living people in the world that evaluated them in terms of lifestyle, diet and their spiritual approach to life. According to the authors of the study, the main determinants of the Okinawans' successful ageing are diet, regular exercise, non-smoking, moderate intake of alcohol and minimal stress.

The Theories of Ageing

An important aspect of the Live-Long Code approach to successful ageing is an understanding of why we age; in other words, we need to know the causes of ageing. This is important because the practices in the Live-Long Code have been formulated in direct response to these causes of ageing. For example, one of the theories of ageing is the free radical theory. This theory claims that free radical damage causes ageing by oxidising the cells in our bodies. The practice to prevent this happening involves a high intake of foods rich in antioxidants and the additional support of our diets with antioxidant supplements. So by understanding the theory of free radical ageing, we are better equipped to implement antidotes to ageing. Armed with this and other correct information, you will be better prepared for guarding against unwanted health issues.

There are ever-increasing numbers of theories around ageing, but currently only five have gained widespread acceptance from the medical community. These are the free radical damage theory, the wear and tear theory, the hormonal theory, the telomere theory and the genetic control theory. Most ageing theories fall into one of two major groups: the group that believes that ageing is primarily caused from within the cells (sometimes referred to as programmed theories) and the group that believes that ageing is caused by random events outside the cells (accidental or damage theories). Proponents of the first broad category contend that we possess genetically pre-programmed biological clocks that instruct our bodies when it is time to start ageing. The second hypothesis contends that extrinsic factors such as stressful environments, pollution and exposure to toxic elements within food and drink cause our bodies to age. The hormonal and telomere theories are examples of programmed theories, while the free radical damage theory can be thought of as containing elements of both hypotheses.

The Live-Long Code considers all these theories to be of interest. The free radical theory and the hormone theory are both very well known in the scientific community and are fundamental to the understanding of anti-ageing medicine. The telomere theory is gathering increased attention and may well offer great promise for the future of anti-ageing medicine. The two other predominant theories are also worth considering.

The Free Radical Damage Theory of Ageing

The free radical damage theory of ageing was developed by Denham Harman MD, a professor at the University of Nebraska, in 1956. This theory has become one of the classic models of ageing. At one stage many researchers believed that this theory explained the fundamental cause of ageing; however, after much study, most would now agree that the oxidative process influences many illnesses associated with ageing but is not the single determinant of the ageing process or of lifespan. Notwithstanding this, the oxidative process has a cumulative effect on health, disease and ageing, and as such it is well worth taking a closer look at the free radical damage theory.

A free radical is an atom, molecule or molecular fragment that contains at least one unpaired electron (in contrast to normal molecules, which contain only paired electrons). Free radicals, together with non-radicals that contribute to free radical production, are often referred to as reactive oxygen species. Free radicals are a by-product of aerobic, or oxygen-using, metabolism that generates ATP, the cell's energy source, from the foods we eat. During this process, which occurs in specialised cell parts called mitochondria, electrons are passed from molecule to molecule. Most of the electrons (97–99 per cent) are taken up by oxygen at the end of the transport chain. The remaining electrons combine incorrectly with oxygen to form superoxide, a free radical that is the major source of other free radicals in the cell. Having an unpaired electron makes a free radical unstable, so it tries to stabilise itself by either gaining an additional electron or losing its unpaired electron. It can only accomplish this by reacting with other cell molecules, such as proteins, lipids and DNA. When the free radical gains or loses an electron, it converts the donor/recipient molecule into a free radical, thus initiating a destructive cascade of free radical reactions.

Free radical reactions cause widespread damage to the cell molecules and, subsequently, the cells themselves. Many of the detrimental effects of free radical reactions occur within the mitochondria, particularly the mitochondrial DNA, which contains the genetic information needed for the production of proteins and other molecules used during energy production. Unlike damage to the DNA of the cell nucleus, damage to mitochondrial DNA is often not repaired. Instead, it accumulates, leading to ever-increasing functional impairment. Other molecules also cease to function normally when damaged by free radical reactions. This in turn disrupts the vital cellular systems that require those molecules for proper functioning. When the damage inflicted by free radical reactions becomes so severe that the cell cannot repair it or compensate for it, the cell dies. If this process occurs in many cells throughout an organ or tissue, the result can be irreversible organ failure. Research has shown that the damaging effects of free radicals on molecular and cellular function are involved not only in ageing, but also in diseases such as atherosclerosis, cancer and Alzheimer's disease.

The body is not defenceless against free radical damage. Many free radicals are detoxified by specialised enzymes and molecules called antioxidants. However, if free radical production is increased and/or antioxidant activity is decreased, the incidence of free radical reactions escalates, with potentially disastrous effects. The free radical damage theory of ageing attributes the ageing process to an imbalance between free radicals and the body's defences against them. The influence of free radicals on disease processes is undoubtedly determined by this relationship as well.

To compensate for the effects of oxidation and free radical damage, nature has designed a sophisticated method to maintain free radical activity by providing naturally occurring antioxidants, substances that work against oxidation and free radical damage by providing donor electrons, thus neutralising free radical activity. This is why most nutritionists will espouse high-antioxidant foods.

The Wear and Tear Theory of Ageing

Dr August Weismann, a German biologist, first formulated this theory in 1882. Weisman is considered to be one of the most important evolutionary biologists of his era. He believed that the body and its cells were damaged by overuse and abuse; that the liver, stomach, kidneys, skin and other organs are worn down by toxins in our diet and in the environment, by the excessive consumption of fat, sugar, caffeine, alcohol and nicotine, by the ultraviolet rays of the sun and by the many other physical and emotional stresses to which we subject our bodies. Wear and tear is not confined to our organs, however; it also takes place on the cellular level.

Of course, even if you've never smoked or drunk alcohol, if you've stayed out of the sun and eaten only natural foods, simply using your body in the act of living still wears it out; as the body ages, our very cells feel the effect, no matter how healthy our lifestyle is. Exposure to 'toxic' elements will just wear it out more quickly.

A younger person's body has its own maintenance and repair system, which helps to compensate for the effects of both normal and excessive wear and tear. With age the body loses its ability to repair the ongoing damage caused by diet, environmental toxins, bacteria or viruses. This is why Weismann believed that older people die of diseases that they could have resisted when they were younger.

The Hormonal Theory of Ageing

The hormonal or neuroendocrine theory of ageing was first proposed by Professor Vladimir Dilman and Ward Dean MD and elaborates on ideas about wear and tear by focusing on the neuroendocrine system. This is a complicated network of biochemicals that controls the release of hormones by a walnut-sized gland in the brain called the hypothalamus.

The hypothalamus controls various elements that instruct other organs and glands when to release their hormones. It also monitors and responds to the body's hormone levels and activity. As we grow older, the hypothalamus loses its precision and the receptors that deal with individual hormones become less sensitive to them. Accordingly, as we age the secretion of many hormones declines and their effectiveness is reduced.

According to the hormonal theory, ageing is a series of 'pauses'. Female menopause reflects a pause in the female endocrine system, while the male andropause reflects a pause in the male endocrine system. Similarly, a pause in the thyroid gland will result in hypothyrodism, and a pause in the pituitary gland will result in a deficiency of growth hormone.

One theory for the loss of regulation in the hypothalamus is that it is damaged over time by the hormone cortisol. Cortisol is produced from the adrenal glands located on the kidneys and is considered to be a 'dark hormone' whose production is increased by stress. It is one of the few hormones whose production increases with age. If cortisol damages the hypothalamus, then over time it creates a vicious cycle of hypothalamic damage, leading to more cortisol production and more hypothalamic damage, and so on and so on. This damage could lead to other hormonal imbalances as the hypothalamus loses its ability to control the endocrine system. According to this theory then, there is a direct link between mental and physical stress and the ageing process.

The hormonal theory of ageing has led to the belief that hormone replacement therapy (HRT) can help the body's hormonal clock to reset itself and thus potentially delay the effects of ageing. This has led to the frequent use of HRT, which is a somewhat controversial practice. This hormone replacement goes beyond the practices commonly used to treat menopausal women. For example, while it is 'normal' for a man in his sixties to produce far less testosterone than he would have in his early twenties, advocates of bio-identical HRT use would argue that restoring these hormone levels to where they were in youthful vigour will bring a host of benefits.

In writing this book I have visited Cenegenics, one of the leading clinics in the field of anti-ageing medicine. Cenegenics brings a multidimensional approach to anti-ageing, which echoes many aspects of the Live-Long Code. At the clinic they provide comprehensive testing of their clients in order to evaluate precisely what their biomarkers of ageing indicate. Then, to help achieve healthy longevity goals, they prescribe a lifestyle based around nutrition, supplementation and exercise choices, and frequently support this by incorporating bio-identical HRT. I believe that hormone replacement using bio-identical hormones offers an interesting avenue for prolonging healthy longevity. However, at this point I don't believe that we have enough information to conclude that HRT is safe enough for all to use, even with medical supervision. The fact is that doctors differ on this subject and until there is broader consensus on its safety, we must wait and see. This technology is still evolving, and in time it may well become an element of the Live-Long Code.

The Telomere Theory of Ageing

The telomere theory of ageing holds great promise for longevity medicine. A telomere is a sequence of amino acids found at the tip of the chromosome of most cells. Studies have shown that with each cell division, the telomere becomes shorter and after approximately 50 replications (known as the Hayflick limit), the telomere is reduced to a mere nub. At this point the cell stops replicating and begins to die.

Current theory declares that genes previously covered by the telomere become exposed and active, producing proteins that trigger the tissue to deteriorate (the beginning of ageing). It has been discovered that sperm cells and cancer cells do not exhibit telomere loss associated with replication and death. Recent research has also revealed that a telomere-preserving enzyme called telomerase has the potential to increase the Hayflick limit. Telomerase therefore appears to repair and replace telomeres, helping to re-regulate the clock that controls the lifespan of dividing cells. Changing or resetting the genetic clock to yield the desired result with reference to anti-ageing may be one of the answers to the question of ageing. Does this suggest that we will see telomerase therapy in the foreseeable future? Perhaps, but current wisdom maintains that methods of reducing and reversing the ageing process that are known at the moment to be reliable should be followed until the science is better understood. We already know that the speed of the genetic clock can be greatly influenced by our lifestyle. For example, DNA is easily oxidised and this damage can be accumulated from diet, toxins, pollution, radiation and other outside influences. Thus, we each have the ability to accelerate DNA damage or slow it down and the Live-Long Code acts to influence this effect and slow down the genetic clock.

The Genetic Control Theory of Ageing

Scientists regard this theory as what they call a 'planned obsolescence' because it focuses on the encoded programming within our DNA. Our DNA is the blueprint of life, obtained from our parents. It means we are born with a unique code and a predetermined tendency to certain types of physical and mental functioning that regulate the rate at which we age. Thus, proponents of the genetic control theory of ageing believe that lifespan is determined by the genes we inherit. Ageing begins at conception. Evidence cited in support of the genetic theory of ageing includes the fact that life expectancy is consistent across members of a species. The fact that females tend to live longer than males is observed among most animal species, not only among humans. We have established that long-lived parents tend to have long-lived children and that some families can be identified as having higher numbers of centenarians. Of course, on the other hand it could be argued that families are more likely to share a common lifestyle, which could account for at least some of these facts.

The genes that positively affect ageing are often called longevity assurance genes. Some such helpful genes include one version of a gene for a protein called apolipoprotein E, as well as certain versions of genes for immune proteins.

Another aspect of the genetic influence on ageing can be seen by looking at our mitochondria, the energy powerhouses of our cells. Mitochondrial gene mutations can result in the loss of the ability to generate energy and can ultimately lead to cell death. Finally, mutations can occur in mitochondrial genes that are associated with Parkinson's and Alzheimer's diseases, both of which are related to ageing.

Even the strongest proponents of the genetic control theory of ageing acknowledge that external influences can affect our genes. Our genetic structure can be modified or damaged by free radicals, toxins and radiation. Recognising the interplay between our genes and the external conditions to which we subject them should lead to a deeper understanding of the ageing process. Therefore, in essence, our genes determine our lifespan. This theory has definite merit; research has established a genetic link to many diseases. In the future, these diseases may be treatable or preventable when we have deciphered our genetic code. Some believe that our lifespan is likely to be 30 per cent determined by our genes and 70 per cent by our lifestyle. Again, until safe drugs are available to alter our genes, the best we can do is practise those lifestyle changes espoused by the Live-Long Code which have been proven to retard genetically linked diseases. Early medical detection for those with a predisposition to genetically linked illness such as Alzheimer's disease and certain types of cancer is a must.

For most of us the ageing process really begins around the age of 30, when the body starts to break down. Prior to this, most of us are still building new tissue. The goal of the Live-Long Code is to slow this breakdown process and reinvigorate your own ability to build tissue. The earlier you start this process, the better; however, it is never too late and people in their sixties and seventies can still benefit significantly from the Live-Long Code.

We know that the major diseases of ageing, such as diabetes, heart disease and cancer, are largely preventable. Thanks to advances in our understanding of medical science, we have the tools to enhance immune function, improve circulation to the brain and heart and generally improve vitality.

As a first step to achieving a healthier and longer life it is useful to have a deeper understanding of your current health status. To achieve this we will use the Live-Long Code Health Profile to monitor your progress towards more youthful ageing. Now let's look at how healthy you really are.

CHAPTER TWO

The Live-Long Code
Health Profile

'How are you?' is a universal greeting to which we most likely respond every day without actually considering the full and true answer. Do we even know the true answer? In this chapter I want to guide you through a health profile that will analyse how you really are and set the foundation stone for the Live-Long Code Programme. This measured approach will not only enable you to answer vital questions about your health, but also begin the journey towards achieving a longer, healthier and happier life. It will enable you to begin setting health goals and to develop a unique personal health plan to reach those goals. It will help you make the best use of the appropriate healthcare professionals. You can reuse this tool at regular intervals to check back and see how you're doing and if you need to adjust your health plan. It is your health, your body and your will.

A healthy lifestyle isn't the sole preserve of the health experts. Good health, wellness and longevity should be for everyone, regardless of social status, personal habits and individual circumstances. The Live-Long Code Health Profile helps you to have a more complete understanding of your current health status. You should update this profile every month to monitor your progress towards better health and longevity.

The Live-Long Code Health Profile combines the wisdom of the East with the best Western health knowledge, together with traditional wisdom and the most cutting-edge medical advances. It also utilises recent developments in scientific health measurements. After completing the test you will have in your armoury a dynamic tool for monitoring and caring for your health. This profile will guide your choices for personal health and well being. The Live-Long Code Health Profile evolves from an extensive, user-friendly gauge of general health that can be easily self-assessed. Despite all the preventative healthcare methods currently available, most people have never before had the means to assess their own health status in such a comprehensive manner and plan a course of action to improve it.

My medical clinic combines the best of conventional medicine with knowledge from the East and I've used my experience and exposure to both medical cultures to create an effective measurement plan. The Live-Long Code Health Profile will become your roadmap and compass, guiding you on a journey to continued good health and successful longevity. The profile is based on a new vision of healthcare, where the focus is on feeling good and on self-enabled health as opposed to illness and reliance on others or the healthcare system.

So What Is Optimal Health and Wellness?

We are all familiar with the phrase 'your health is your wealth'. It is true that good health is a basic requirement for enjoyable everyday living. It should be your number one goal, on a day-to-day basis, throughout your life. It should be your constant goal even if you are enjoying good health today. If you were going to buy a car and learned that a particular model was very unreliable and would break down regularly, you would undoubtedly be put off buying it. The government, in fact, insists that we check our cars to ensure that they are roadworthy and a car that does not pass this test must be taken off the road until it satisfies accepted standards. It would seem silly if the government worked the other way round and insisted on a car roadworthy test after every car crash, and yet that is precisely the approach we take when it comes to our health – we often only think about and evaluate our health *after* we have crashed. Surely it makes sense to switch the emphasis to promotion of health and prevention of illness rather than on sickness itself.

Unfortunately, many people continue to die prematurely or live with a constant struggle with poor health, disability or disease. Some don't seek medical advice or obtain treatment when they need it, or don't get the help they need even when they look for it; others simply do not know that many diseases, injuries and illnesses are preventable. But why do we put up with being sick if we don't have to?

Good health relies upon a number of factors: the personal and genetic traits that you have inherited from your parents, the environment in which you live and work, your personal habits and lifestyle choices and the care you have received from healthcare professionals. All of these affect health. Of all these factors it is the one over which you have direct control over that is probably the most influential with regard to your health – your lifestyle choices. Many of us fail to see that there are actions we can take ourselves to maintain and improve our health, but there are serious risks stemming from personal habits – your lifestyle – that you can control. Most health experts now agree that lifestyle is the most important factor affecting your health and quality of life. In fact, it is estimated that the risks associated with seven of the 10 leading causes of death could be reduced through common-sense changes in lifestyle. Your Live-Long Code Health Profile provides the compass to making these changes.

Health is about far more than the absence of disease and disability. In addition to complete physical and mental well-being, health also means achieving a satisfying and peaceful life. You yourself are responsible for adding quality to your life. Positive approaches and raised awareness, combined with healthy social practices and environment, can all make a spectacular difference. You have the opportunity to change when you recognise that the combination of your habits, emotional and psychological state, social situation, personality and character affects your health and how you feel every day.

Simply put, for optimal health and well being, knowledge is the key. To be at your healthiest, you must identify and realise your health and wellness goals. It may well be that to do this you will have to change or find ways to cope with your personal situation.

Of course, there will always be some factors beyond our control, but it will surprise you how many factors you can in fact influence. When you have the information from your Live-Long Code Health Profile, as well as the knowledge and resources that enable you to change, you can improve your health, your well-being and indeed your whole quality of life.

Many healthcare professionals, too, are starting to look beyond diseases, disabilities and symptoms and are starting to help their patients face their health challenges in the 'big picture' context of their overall quality of life. As a result, both professionals and patients now tend to make wiser and more cost-effective choices in the use of healthcare resources.

Designed to help you find or keep good health, the Live-Long Code Health Profile is a tool you can use easily and share with friends and family. Who wouldn't want to see loved ones, friends and family enjoy better health too? Wellness is contagious; if we see a fit, healthy person, we may be inspired to change. Businesses benefit from a healthier workforce, and society benefits as a whole, with less strain being placed on the health service. People who focus on wellness instead of illness spend far less time and money going for medical help, which leaves costly healthcare resources for the people who truly need them. As parents, when you set an example of leading a healthier and more fulfilled life, your children benefit directly and learn how to create their own good health habits. Eventually, as your children grow into adults, this new approach to health will become part of their lives, and gradually a new optimum-health culture will become a reality.

Taking Charge of Your Personal Health

Taking care of yourself starts with the ability to view personal health from a holistic – 'whole story' – viewpoint. It includes identifying self-care resources; being willing to participate in making health decisions when choices arise; and having the knowledge, ability and determination to practise disease prevention. More than that, practising self-care usually means improving your living conditions and your lifestyle; making wise use of self-care products and technology; using mind and body health-enhancing techniques such as yoga and chi kung; and taking into account how your personal attitudes and beliefs affect your health.

In medical practices today there has developed an overreliance on drugs by both doctors and healthcare consumers. It is this 'silver bullet' approach that has resulted in the increasing number of cases of antibiotic-resistant infections. My professor of traditional Chinese medicine had an interesting way of putting it; he believes that overuse of antibiotics is like discharging a shotgun every time you hear a noise in your house. It's true that occasionally there may be an invader, but the damage caused by the deterrent is often more harmful. In the same way that having a secure lock on your door makes more sense than using a shotgun, a better approach to health is preventative. Medical science and technology, which have in other ways so much to be proud of, have encouraged people to hand over responsibility for their personal health to 'the experts' and to what they consider to be quick fixes for their problems. People practising self-care know the appropriate actions when it comes to disease, symptoms and injury prevention, and are able to cope much more satisfactorily with minor illnesses. They are more aware of their health and know when it is appropriate to seek help. This knowledge and having the tools to take an active, well-informed and hands-on role is crucial to becoming healthier and eventually reaching the goal of peak health.

The Live-Long Code Health Profile is a powerful tool to assist you in identifying and assessing your health requirements so that you can make wiser choices for enhancing your health. Your Live-Long Code Health Profile has long-term, ongoing benefits in that it can be used regularly and indefinitely to examine your health status. At any point you can go back to it to take another look at your personal health to target areas that need enhancement. This gives you a meaningful way to zero in on your existing health weaknesses in order to face future health challenges. Your profile provides you with a measuring stick and gives understandable and unbiased information.

Approaching health as a dynamic and variable condition where you, the individual, have a great deal of control can be both motivating and empowering. Such a drastic mental shift is bound to lead to better outcomes in the general health of individuals, and ultimately in the health of society at large. If you make the commitment, you will be able to answer that daily question very honestly and very optimistically: 'I'm very well, thank you.'

The Live-Long Code Health Profile: Measuring Your Health

The Live-Long Code Health Profile encompasses a broad spectrum and measures both your current health condition and the ways in which you can change it, when necessary, with positive health action. It will provide a clear picture of your current benchmark of general health. Although the questions are designed to apply to the widest possible segment of society, some of them may not be applicable if you have chronic diseases or disabilities. If this applies to you, you can still take the test, but you may need to seek further guidance from your doctors or other healthcare professionals. You may also find my previous book, *The Healing Code*, a useful tool in your health recovery.

All of us want good health, but many of us do not know how to be as healthy as possible. Good health is not a matter of chance; you have to work at it. The time you take to complete this survey may help you add years to your life! You may well identify aspects of your way of life that are risky to your health. This information can help you pinpoint the dangers and amend them to create a new, healthier lifestyle, which means that you may well start to feel better, look better and live longer. Remember, this is not a pass-or-fail exam. Its purpose is simply to tell you what you need to do to stay healthy or become healthier.

Self-Test Health Measurements

Self-Test One: Blood Pressure

High blood pressure puts you at greater risk for heart disease. Your blood pressure is made up of two numbers, the systolic number (the first number when your blood pressure is measured, which represents the pressure when the heart beats) and diastolic number (the second number in your blood pressure measure, representing the pressure when the heart rests). If one or both of these numbers are high, you have high blood pressure. One in three adults has high blood pressure, and nearly one-third of them don't know they have it. Most pharmacies will check your blood pressure, and blood pressure monitors are relatively inexpensive to buy and are available from www.immortalitycode.com.

Category	Systolic (top number)	Diastolic (bottom number)
Normal	Less than 120	Less than 80
Prehypertension	120–139	80–89
High blood pressure		
Stage 1	140–159	90–99
Stage 2	160 or higher	100 or higher

Score Box			
Date	Result	Date	Result

Self-Test Two: Body Mass Index

The body mass index (BMI) became popular during the early 1980s as obesity started to become an issue. BMI is a relationship between your height and weight and provides a simple numeric measure of a person's 'thickness'. It is just intended to be used as a simple means of classifying individuals with an average body composition. A frequent use of BMI is to assess how much an individual's body weight departs from what is 'normal' or desirable for a person of his or her height. The weight excess or deficiency may, in part, be accounted for by body fat, although other factors such as muscularity also affect BMI. BMI levels for overweight and obesity are now set by the World Health Organization (WHO), which defines 'overweight' as a BMI equal to or more than 25, and 'obesity' as a BMI equal to or more than 30.

Note that BMI doesn't take into account body composition; therefore it may give misleading readings and overestimate body fat in athletes and other people who have a very muscular build. It may also underestimate body fat in people who have lost muscle mass.

	BMI
Underweight	Below 18.5
Normal	18.5–24.9
Overweight	25.0–29.9
Obesity	30.0–39.9
Extreme obesity	40.0 and above

Score Box			
Date	Result	Date	Result

Self-Test Three: Waist Measurement

Waist measurements are a good indicator of abdominal fat, which is a predictor of a person's chances of developing risk factors for heart disease and other diseases.

Measure your waist at the top of your hipbones, where it is narrowest. A woman with a waist measurement of greater than 35 inches runs a higher risk of developing heart disease and other diseases. A man with a waist measurement of greater than 40 inches runs a higher risk for developing heart disease and other diseases.

Score Box			
Date	Result	Date	Result

Self-Test Four: Body Fat Percentage

Body fat percentage can be determined by hand-held devices, underwater weighing and skin fold callipers. If you are a member of a gym they should be able to help you with this calculation. Otherwise many pharmacies have devices to give you this calculation.

	Age	Underfat	Healthy	Overfat	Obese
Female	20–39	5–20	21–33	34–38	> 38
	40–59	5–22	23–34	35–40	> 40
	60–79	5–23	24–36	37–41	> 41
Male	20–39	5–7	8–20	21–25	> 25
	40–59	5–10	11–21	22–27	> 27
	60–79	5–12	13–25	26–30	> 30

International BMI Table

WEIGHT		HEIGHT IN FEET/INCHES AND METRES											
LB	KG	4'8" 1.42 m	4'10" 1.47 m	5'0" 1.52 m	5'2" 1.57 m	5'4" 1.63 m	5'6" 1.68 m	5'8" 1.73 m	5'10" 1.78 m	6'0" 1.83 m	6'2" 1.88 m	6'4" 1.93 m	6'6" 1.98 m
100	45.4	22.4	20.9	19.5	18.3	17.2	16.1	15.2	14.3	13.6	12.8	12.2	11.6
105	47.6	23.5	21.9	20.5	19.2	18.0	16.9	16.0	15.1	14.2	13.5	12.8	12.1
110	49.9	24.7	23.0	21.5	20.1	18.9	17.8	16.7	15.8	14.9	14.1	13.4	12.7
115	52.2	25.8	24.0	22.5	21.0	19.7	18.6	17.5	16.5	15.6	14.8	14.0	13.3
120	54.4	26.9	25.1	23.4	21.9	20.6	19.4	18.2	17.2	16.3	15.4	14.6	13.9
125	56.7	28.0	26.1	24.4	22.9	21.5	20.2	19.0	17.9	17.0	16.0	15.2	14.4
130	59.0	29.1	27.2	25.4	23.8	22.3	21.0	19.8	18.7	17.6	16.7	15.8	15.0
135	61.2	30.3	28.2	26.4	24.7	23.2	21.8	20.5	19.4	18.3	17.3	16.4	15.6
140	63.5	31.4	29.3	27.3	25.6	24.0	22.6	21.3	20.1	19.0	18.0	17.0	16.2
145	65.8	32.5	30.3	28.3	26.5	24.9	23.4	22.0	20.8	19.7	18.6	17.6	16.8
150	68.0	33.6	31.3	29.3	27.4	25.7	24.2	22.8	21.5	20.3	19.3	18.3	17.3
155	70.3	34.7	32.4	30.3	28.3	26.6	25.0	23.6	22.2	21.0	19.9	18.9	17.9
160	72.6	35.9	33.4	31.2	29.3	27.5	25.8	24.3	23.0	21.7	20.5	19.5	18.5
165	74.8	37.0	34.5	32.2	30.2	28.3	26.6	25.1	23.7	22.4	21.2	20.1	19.1
170	77.1	38.1	35.5	33.2	31.1	29.2	27.4	25.8	24.4	23.1	21.8	20.7	19.6
175	79.4	39.2	36.6	34.2	32.0	30.0	28.2	26.6	25.1	23.7	22.5	21.3	20.2
180	81.6	40.4	37.6	35.2	32.9	30.9	29.1	27.4	25.8	24.4	23.1	21.9	20.8
185	83.9	41.5	38.7	36.1	33.8	31.8	29.9	28.1	26.5	25.1	23.8	22.5	21.4
190	86.2	42.6	39.7	37.1	34.8	32.6	30.7	28.9	27.3	25.8	24.4	23.1	22.0
195	88.5	43.7	40.8	38.1	35.7	33.5	31.5	29.6	28.0	26.4	25.0	23.7	22.5
200	90.7	44.8	41.8	39.1	36.6	34.3	32.3	30.4	28.7	27.1	25.7	24.3	23.1
205	93.0	46.0	42.8	40.0	37.5	35.2	33.1	31.2	29.4	27.8	26.3	25.0	23.7

LB	KG	4'8" 1.42 m	4'10" 1.47 m	5'0" 1.52 m	5'2" 1.57 m	5'4" 1.63 m	5'6" 1.68 m	5'8" 1.73 m	5'10" 1.78 m	6'0" 1.83 m	6'2" 1.88 m	6'4" 1.93 m	6'6" 1.98 m
230	104.3	51.6	48.1	44.9	42.1	39.5	37.1	35.0	33.0	31.2	29.5	28.0	26.6
235	106.6	52.7	49.1	45.9	43.0	40.3	37.9	35.7	33.7	31.9	30.2	28.6	27.2
240	108.9	53.8	50.2	46.9	43.9	41.2	38.7	36.5	34.4	32.5	30.8	29.2	27.7
245	111.1	54.9	51.2	47.8	44.8	42.1	39.5	37.3	35.2	33.2	31.5	29.8	28.3
250	113.4	56.0	52.2	48.8	45.7	42.9	40.3	38.0	35.9	33.9	32.1	30.4	28.9
255	115.7	57.2	53.3	49.8	46.6	43.8	41.2	38.8	36.6	34.6	32.7	31.0	29.5
260	117.9	58.3	54.3	50.8	47.5	44.6	42.0	39.5	37.3	35.3	33.4	31.6	30.0
265	120.4	59.4	55.4	51.7	48.5	45.5	42.8	40.3	38.0	35.9	34.0	32.3	30.6
270	122.5	60.5	56.4	52.7	49.4	46.3	43.6	41.0	38.7	36.6	34.7	32.9	31.2
280	127.0	62.8	58.5	54.7	51.2	48.1	45.2	42.6	40.2	38.0	35.9	34.1	32.4
285	129.3	63.9	59.6	55.7	52.1	48.9	46.0	43.3	40.9	38.6	36.6	34.7	32.9
290	131.5	65.0	60.6	56.6	53.0	49.8	46.8	44.1	41.6	39.3	37.2	35.3	33.5
295	133.8	66.1	61.6	57.6	54.0	50.6	47.6	44.8	42.3	40.0	37.9	35.9	34.1
300	136.1	67.3	62.7	58.6	54.9	51.5	48.4	45.6	43.0	40.7	38.5	36.5	34.7
305	138.3	68.4	63.7	59.6	55.8	52.3	49.2	46.4	43.8	41.4	39.2	37.1	35.2
310	140.6	69.5	64.8	60.5	56.7	53.2	50.0	47.1	44.5	42.0	39.8	37.7	35.8
315	142.9	70.6	65.8	61.5	57.6	54.1	50.8	47.9	45.2	42.7	40.4	38.3	36.4
320	145.1	71.7	66.9	62.5	58.5	54.9	51.6	48.7	45.9	43.4	41.1	38.9	37.0
325	147.4	72.9	67.9	63.5	59.4	55.8	52.5	49.4	46.6	44.1	41.7	39.6	37.6
330	149.7	74.0	69.0	64.4	60.4	56.6	53.3	50.2	47.3	44.8	42.4	40.2	38.1
335	152.0	75.1	70.0	65.4	61.3	57.5	54.1	50.9	48.1	45.4	43.0	40.8	38.7
340	154.2	76.2	71.1	66.4	62.2	58.4	54.9	51.7	48.8	46.1	43.6	41.4	39.3
345	156.5	77.3	72.1	67.4	63.1	59.2	55.7	52.5	49.5	46.8	44.3	42.0	39.9
350	158.8	78.5	73.1	68.3	64.0	60.1	56.5	53.2	50.2	47.5	44.9	42.6	40.4

HEIGHT IN FEET/INCHES AND METRES

WEIGHT

Score Box			
Date	Result	Date	Result

Self-Test Five: One-Mile Walk

A timed one-mile walk is a good method of determining your fitness level. James Rippe MD has developed age-specific data for a flat one-mile test. Make sure you warm up for five minutes first and stretch, then walk the mile as quickly as you can without running out of steam.

Age	Time Acceptable
Under 30	13 minutes
30–39	14 minutes
40–49	14 minutes 42 seconds
50–69	15 minutes
70 or over	18 minutes 18 seconds

If you achieve the time for your age group by less than three minutes, you are in good shape. If you exceed the time by more than three minutes, you're not in the best shape aerobically. Either way, don't worry, just keep walking!

Score Box			
Date	Result	Date	Result

Self-Test Six: Cholesterol Levels

Cholesterol is made up of two components, LDL ('bad' cholesterol) and HDL ('good' cholesterol). When you have your cholesterol tested, you will see 'total cholesterol', which is the sum of all the cholesterol in your blood. The higher your total cholesterol, the greater your risk for heart disease. You will also see a listing of HDL cholesterol. Higher levels of HDL are associated with improved heart health because HDL carries the bad cholesterol back to the liver and helps prevent it from building up on the walls of the arteries.

Self-testing cholesterol kits are available in most pharmacies and from www.immortalitycode.com.

National Cholesterol Education Programme
Cholesterol Guidelines

	Desirable	Borderline High	High
Total cholesterol	Less than 200	200–239	240 and higher
LDL cholesterol (the 'bad' cholesterol)	Less than 130	130–159	160 and higher
HDL cholesterol (the 'good' cholesterol)	50 and higher	40–49	Less than 40
Triglycerides	Less than 200	200–399	400 and higher

Score Box

Date	Result	Date	Result

Self-Test Seven: Blood Glucose Levels

Blood glucose level tests measure the amount of glucose in your blood. You need a certain amount of glucose in your blood, but too much is a bad thing. Diabetes is a disease in which blood glucose levels are above normal.

There are several tests used to determine if a person is diabetic. The numbers that represent an unhealthy amount of glucose in your blood are dependent on the test taken (fasting plasma glucose test, oral glucose tolerance test or random plasma glucose test). Blood glucose level tests are available in most pharmacies and from www. immortalitycode.com.

If you are 45 or older, you should consider getting tested for diabetes. If you are 45 or older and overweight, it is strongly recommended that you get tested. Signs of diabetes include being very thirsty, urinating often, feeling very hungry or tired, losing weight without trying, sores that heal slowly, dry, itchy skin, losing the feeling in your feet or having tingling in your feet, or having blurry eyesight. However, although you may have one or more of these signs, you may have had no signs at all and still have pre-diabetes or diabetes. A blood test to check your glucose levels will determine this.

Score Box			
Date	Result	Date	Result

Self-Test Eight: Balance Test

There is a close relationship between balance, memory and reaction speed. Loss of balance is a sign of ageing and can seriously impinge on quality of life. To perform the test, raise one leg out in front with your knee bent at a right angle. You can stretch your arms out to the sides to help you balance. Close your eyes and see how long it takes before you have to put your foot down or open your eyes to regain your balance. Get someone to time you.

Time in Seconds	Age Rating
More than 30	20
21–30	30
16–20	40
10–15	50
Less than 10	60

Score Box			
Date	Result	Date	Result

Self-Test Nine: Reaction Speed Test

Humans automatically respond to physical occurrences or stimuli. Reactions are usually caused by something physical like pressure, sound or pain. The body has sense organs that pick up this information – this is what is classed as a reaction.

What is the reaction process in our bodies?

- Firstly, you see an image with your eyes.
- This image is then stored in your retina.
- The message is then sent to the visual cortex in your brain.
- That sends a message telling your body, your arms and your legs to move.

There is a simple test you can do with a ruler. Get someone to hold a ruler above your hand and drop it without telling you. The aim is for you to catch the ruler before it drops past your hands onto the floor. Position your open hand 10 cm (4 in) below the bottom of the ruler. When your partner drops the ruler, grab it as quickly as possible. If you catch it, note by looking at the measurement markings how far down the ruler you caught it.

What is the average reaction time for a human being?
A good response would be 180 milliseconds (0.18 seconds). However, the average is around 250 milliseconds (0.25 seconds).

Distance	Age Rating
Less than 10cm (4in)	20
15cm (6in)	25
20cm (8in)	30
25cm (10in)	35
30cm (12in) or miss	40+

Score Box			
Date	Result	Date	Result

Self-Test Ten: Upper Body Strength Test

Maintaining strong muscles is an important way to stay young and fit. As we age we lose muscle mass and consequently muscle function. This push-up test measures your upper body strength. Men should use a standard push-up position with the knees straight and the hands and toes touching the floor. Women may do push-ups from the bent-knee position.

Bend from the elbow until the chest is about 3in from the floor.

Extend arms back to the start. Do as many push-ups as possible without stopping, counting the total.

Score/Age	21–30yrs	31–40yrs	41–50yrs	51–60yrs	61–70yrs
Excellent	50+	40+	35+	30+	25+
Very good	39–49	35–39	30–34	25–29	20–24
Good	30–38	25–34	21–29	18–24	17–19
Average	17–29	13–24	11–20	9–17	6–16
Poor	4–16	2–12	1–10	1–8	1–5
Very poor	0–3	0–1	0	0	0

Score Box			
Date	Result	Date	Result

Self-Test Eleven: Flexibility Test

Flexibility is another thing that usually deteriorates as we get older, but good flexibility is essential for injury prevention. The movement restrictions that we associate with ageing can be prevented or minimised by maintaining good flexibility. Having the right balance between flexibility and good posture will ensure that you retain youthful movement and dexterity.

The test for flexibility that we will use is called the trunk flexibility test. Warm up your hamstrings prior to the test.

- Sit upright with your feet flat against a wall.
- Reach forward and try to touch the wall.
- Get someone to measure the distance between your fingertips and the wall.

Excellent	Palms on wall
Good	Fingertips on wall
Average	1–12 cm away
Poor	Greater than 12 cm away

Score Box			
Date	Result	Date	Result

Self-Test Twelve: Heart Rate Test

The resting heart rate of different individuals varies significantly. Generally, people with better cardiovascular health have lower heart rates. Although resting heart rate usually increases with age, very high (above 101) or very low (below 50) resting heart rates may indicate that something is wrong. To determine your true resting heart rate, test it first thing in the morning before you get out of bed. If your heart rate is elevated in the mornings or if it seems unnaturally high during exercise, then you should speak to your doctor about it.

The ideal place to count your pulse is at the radial arteries on the wrist. Place your index and middle finger lightly over one of these arteries and, with a watch in hand, count the beats for 60 seconds.

Beats per Minute	Age Rating
60	20
65	30
70	40
75	50
80+	60

Score Box			
Date	Result	Date	Result

Self-Test Thirteen: Level of Stress

To determine your current stress level, here is a simple life-stress test that you can take on your own. It is based on internal and external stress factors that affect our daily lives to give your personal stress level.

The following scale was developed by Holmes and Rahe to investigate the relationship between social readjustment, stress and susceptibility to illness. They found that a person with a score of 200–250 during a one-year period has a 50 per cent chance of developing illness or a change in health. With a score of 300 or more, a person's chances increase to 80 per cent. Look over the events listed below and place a check next to it if it has happened to you within the past 12 months.

1. Death of a spouse (100)
2. Divorce (72)
3. Marital separation (65)
4. Death of a close family member (63)
5. Personal injury or illness (53)
6. Marriage (50)
7. Marital reconciliation (45)
8. Change in health of family member (44)
9. Pregnancy (40)
10. Gain of new family member (39)

11. Job change (38)
12. Change in financial status (37)
13. Death of a close friend (36)
14. Increase in arguments with significant other (35)
15. Mortgage or loan of major purchase (home, etc.) (31)
16. Foreclosure of mortgage or loan (30)
17. Change in responsibilities of your job (29)
18. Son or daughter leaving home (29)
19. Trouble with in-laws (29)
20. Outstanding personal achievement (28)
21. Spouse begins or stops work outside the home (26)
22. Revision of personal habits (24)
23. Trouble with boss (23)
24. Change in work hours or conditions (20)
25. Change in residence (20)
26. Change in sleeping habits (16)
27. Change in eating habits (15)
28. Holidays (13)
29. Christmas (12)
30. Minor violations of the law (11)

Total: _____

Interpretation: Drs Holmes and Rahe have shown the relation-ship between recent life changes (exposure to stressors) and future illness. Listed below are the score categories and the related prob-ability of illness for a person in that range. It is estimated that it will take one year to replenish the energy expended in adjusting to any of the changes described in the scale.

0–149	No significant problem	
150–199	Mild stress	35% chance of illness
200–299	Moderate stress	50% chance of illness
300+	Major stress	80% chance of illness

Score Box			
Date	Result	Date	Result

In addition to the Live-Long Code Health Profile, I'd like to bring to your attention a number of blood tests which I recommend that you have on a regular basis. Seek your doctor's guidance, but be aware that these tests can forewarn you of disease before it happens so that you can take preventative action in advance.

If you do take these tests I suggest that you record your results here so that you can keep a record of your progress with these biomarkers from year to year.

Medical Blood Tests

Annual blood testing is one of the most important steps you can take to help prevent life-threatening disease. Armed with your blood test results, you can catch critical changes in your body before they ever manifest as illnesses such as diabetes, heart disease and cancer. Having these tests can empower you to implement a science-based prevention programme that could add decades of healthy life to your personal lifespan.

Most annual medical check-ups include only routine blood tests, if any at all. Far too often, this basic blood work does not test for important markers of disease risk. As a result of failing to analyse blood for proven markers of disease risk, you needlessly expose yourself to the dangers of serious illness.

Below we will discuss the most important tests that people over the age of 40 should have every year. Armed with these results, you can work with the Live-Long Code Programme together with your doctor to avert serious health problems and achieve optimal health.

Medical Test One: Complete Blood Count (CBC)

A complete blood count is the starting point for disease prevention testing. This relatively cheap test gives you and your doctor a snapshot of your overall health, as it provides a broad range of information with which to assess your organ and blood cell status. The CBC measures the number, variety, concentration and quality of red and white blood cells and platelets. This is a useful test to screen for infections, anaemia and other blood abnormalities.

The CBC gives information on the functioning of your cardiovascular system by testing for total cholesterol, HDL (good cholesterol) and LDL (bad cholesterol). The CBC also measures blood glucose, which is a critical marker for detecting diabetes and coronary artery disease. Given that diabetes is on the increase, monitoring these glucose levels is an important preventative step to take. Also included in the CBC is a test for mineral deficiencies such as iron, potassium and calcium.

Medical Test Two: Fibrinogen

Fibrinogen assists in the process of blood clotting, and levels of it in your body rise when there is inflammation present. As heart disease and arthrosclerosis are inflammatory diseases, increased fibrinogen levels are indicative of a potential risk of heart disease or stroke.

High fibrinogen levels are also indicative of other inflammatory disorders such as rheumatoid arthritis. A recent Greek study found an association between higher fibrinogen levels and the occurrence of multiple coronary lesions in patients who had suffered an acute myocardial infarction or heart attack.

A combination of lifestyle and behavioural changes will help lower your fibrinogen levels to an optimum range.

Medical Test Three: Prostate Specific Antigen (PSA)

PSA is a protein produced by the prostate gland in men. Elevated PSA levels could suggest an enlarged prostate, prostate inflammation or sometimes prostate cancer.

It is recommended that men over the age of 50 should have annual PSA tests. If you are at higher risk, for example if you know you have a genetic predisposition towards prostate cancer, then you should probably commence testing in your early forties.

Medical Test Four: Homocysteine

The amino acid homocysteine is produced in the body during the metabolism of methionine. A high homocysteine level has been associated with an increased risk of heart attack and bone fracture as well as a number of other conditions.

A US study tracked 14,916 healthy male doctors with no history of heart disease and found that high homocysteine levels were associated with an almost 300 per cent increase in heart attack risk over a five-year period.

High homocysteine levels combined with low vitamin B12 levels have been linked to an increased risk of bone fracture. A Dutch study indicated that elevated homocysteine levels are also associated with prolonged lower cognitive performance.

Implementing the Live-Long Code Programme can help to optimise homocysteine levels. You may also consider discussing with your doctor the use of vitamins B6 and B12, together with folic acid and trimethylglycine.

Medical Test Five: Thyroid Stimulating Hormone (TSH)

TSH controls thyroid hormone secretion. Low TSH levels indicate hyperthyroidism, or an overactive thyroid, and high levels suggest hypothyroidism, or an underactive thyroid. If a mild version of either of these conditions is not diagnosed it can progress to clinical disease states, where it is often more dangerous. People with severe hypothyroidism and elevated cholesterol levels have an increased risk of atherosclerosis.

Mild hypothyroidism could be a sign of high blood cholesterol, cognitive dysfunction, fatigue, depression or weight gain. Mild hyperthyroidism is often associated with a disturbance in heart rhythm, reduced bone mineral density, weight loss, insomnia, muscle weakness, shortness of breath and heart palpitations.

Measuring TSH is the best test we have for assessing thyroid function and it's recommended that you begin testing TSH at 40 and repeat the test every five years. Natural therapies may help support thyroid health and optimise TSH levels.

Yearly blood testing is a simple and effective way to proactively take charge of your health. A well-chosen selection of blood tests is an excellent complement to the Live-Long Code Programme, as it helps to detect any early warning signs to predict the development of diseases. Many diseases are treatable when caught early enough, but can take hold and severely damage the quality of your life if they go undetected. Identifying these hidden risks will enable you to implement the powerful strategies included in the Live-Long Code, such as weight loss, exercise, supplements and early medication, in order to prevent progression of the illness. Armed with information from these tests on important health biomarkers, you and your doctor can plan and execute a strategy to help you achieve and maintain vibrant good health.

	Current Date	+6 months	+6 months	+6 months	+6 months	+6 months
	Score	Score	Score	Score	Score	Score
BP						
BMI						
Waist						
Body Fat (%)						
One-Mile Walk						
Cholesterol						
Blood glucose						
Balance						
Reactions						
Strength						
Flexibility						
Heart rate						
Stress						
CBC*						
Fibrinogen*						
PSA**						
Homocysteine**						
TSH**						

* Perform these tests every two years.   **Perform these test every five years.

In Summary

- The Live-Long Code Health Profile is a practical tool to use for evaluating your current state of health and to monitor your health progression.
- This tool assists you in taking a hands-on approach to your own health and enables you to take greater responsibility for the management of your health.
- Good self-care requires sound knowledge of your health, lifestyle and other issues revealed in your Live-Long Code Health Profile. This knowledge gives you a broader understanding of your health and particular health improvement needs.
- If you are used to relying on the healthcare system, becoming directly involved in in-depth monitoring of your own health may seem like a radical change. In fact, it is empowering to take control of your personal health destiny.
- Your ongoing success with the Live-Long Code Programme will depend largely on your own personal commitment, which is assisted by continuous evaluation of your health.

You should now have a comprehensive understanding of your current health profile. You are now ready to make changes that will push you towards the best health of your life. I firmly believe that good health begins in a place where people often forget to look – in the mind. So where better to begin our journey than with a question: what is the mind of the immortal?

CHAPTER THREE

The Immortal Mind

Throughout this book we will examine the ageing process and all the factors that contribute to it. We will look at nutrition, genetics, exercise and lifestyle choices that can slow or even reverse the ageing process. However, the most powerful anti-ageing weapon in your arsenal is your mind.

Many studies have proven that our health is greatly affected by our response to stressful life events and in particular our mental reaction to such situations. Many of us believe that the person we are is very much down to our experiences, but this is only half the truth. We are who we are because of the *perception* of our experiences. In other words, the same good and bad things can happen to a number of people but the way they react and respond might be completely different.

A recent study showed that successful athletes tend to have an inbuilt reaction to stressful situations that is likely to support superior performance. The athletes in the study were placed in a powerful MRI brain scanner and shown images of horrific situations, which would typically elicit a stress response. However, something curious was observed. With most people, the area of the brain responsible for stress would become very active on being shown these images, but with the athletes it was the area of the brain responsible for pleasure that showed the most amount of activity. When asked about this, the high-performing athletes said that when they saw the images, while they were initially repelled, they then experienced feelings of gratitude that their lives were much more fortunate than those of the people they were observing.

It seems clear, therefore, that the brain can react in many different ways to stressful situations. Setbacks at work, conflicts with family members, the loss of a loved one – all of these can have a significant impact on our mental state and consequently on our health. However, we can develop and change our reactions so as to create a more positive and healthy response. Committing to a positive attitude towards life and, more importantly, learning how to create it is a key element of the Live-Long Code's approach to making you younger, reducing your biological age and improving your ability to maintain a vigorous and energetic lifestyle.

How Stress Affects Our Longevity

Stress has an impact on both the mind and body, in a variety of ways, and it is pervasive – almost every organ in the body reacts to stress.

The pituitary gland produces an increased amount of the hormone adrenocorticotropic (ACTH), which results in an increased release of the hormones cortisone and cortisol. This increase suppresses the immune function and inhibits our ability to fight disease. These physical changes are a result of the fight-or-flight response, which is designed to help us to react quickly to and deal with immediately threatening situations by allowing the body to produce energy fast in order to react quickly to physical danger. The fight-or-flight response causes the body to excrete amino acids and minerals that support the body's defence mode.

In the modern world our stresses are more likely to be psychological than physical, but the body still responds in the same way. Unfortunately, many people are constantly exposed to psychological stressors and so find themselves trapped in a constant fight-or-flight response state. In this state the body is less efficient at absorbing digestive nutrients; often more gastric acid is produced, and the bowels and intestines may also be adversely affected. Many disorders can result from prolonged stress exposure, and this can result in nutritional deficiencies and impinge on the proper functioning of the nervous system.

Live-Long Code Mind Programme – Introduction

Stress kills; therefore stress reduction prolongs life. About 60 years ago Dr Hans Selye recognised the way in which the stress response affects the body. He noticed that many of his patients had similarities in their psychological and physiological behaviour, including loss of appetite and increased blood pressure. By performing animal studies Selye established that rats exhibited the same physical responses when they were put under stress. Seyle's conclusion was that stress is a non-specific response of the body to any demand placed upon it. More importantly, Seyle also concluded that it is not stress that harms us, but rather the manner in which we respond.

Dr Seyle referred to our response to stress as General Adaptation Syndrome (GAS). This consists of three different stages: alarm, resistance and exhaustion. The alarm stage is the fight-or-flight response we have previously looked at, during which the body releases cortisol and prepares either to confront whatever is threatening us or to retreat hastily from it.

The next stage is resistance, which enables our bodies to adjust to counteract the physiological changes that have occurred in response to the stress. If during this phase the stress does not disappear, the third stage occurs: exhaustion. It is during this phase that the body creates a situation of distress. The response can range from extreme fatigue to disease and possibly even death.

Many modern scientific researchers now believe what traditional Chinese doctors have recognised for thousands of years – that stress contributes to the majority of our major illnesses, including cardiovascular and metabolic diseases, skin disorders and infectious ailments of all kinds, and cancer. Stress is also usually involved in psychological difficulties such as depression and anxiety.

Stress and Ageing

Stress is a normal part of the human condition; any situation, physical or emotional, that causes a bodily response is considered to be stress. So a slight change in temperature causes the body to respond by raising or lowering body temperature and can be called a stress. Even pleasurable experiences such as falling in love, watching an exciting movie or playing a game of tennis are forms of stress.

Pressure at work, relationship and family problems, financial difficulties and getting ready for holidays are sources of stress for many people. Other less obvious forms of stress include everyday encounters with crowds and traffic, starting a career and taking a new job. The state of stress in our body is magnified if we are overworked or lacking in proper sleep, as well as if we are suffering physical illnesses. Some people can comfortably deal with stress in a creative way and take things in their stride; others are more negatively affected by it.

Stress only becomes negative because of our response to it. If your reaction to a big family get-together is anxiety rather than pleasure, your body will react with headaches or digestive issues. It is likely that your immune system will be affected as well.

Negative stress creates a large number of ailments, from anxiety and depression to headaches, fatigue, allergies and loss of appetite, ulcers, high blood pressure and heart disease. In the long run, negative responses have a detrimental effect on the immune system and potentially lead to a variety of neurological conditions, cancers and other diseases typically associated with ageing.

Defeating Stress

There is a growing tendency for people to experience stress and anxiety disorders; disorders characterised by constant worry, insomnia, fatigue and a general feeling of unease. This has also been associated with an increased risk of heart disease. Social and cultural factors greatly influence this phenomenon. Working through lunch, taking less time off and fewer holidays, and generally working harder and spending less time looking after yourself are frequently held up as good examples of how to live with determination and ambition. In addition to this, our world has become more fast paced. We are bombarded with information. The mobile phone and the internet put us permanently in 'on' mode. And with today's round-the-clock access to news – most of which is bad – we are kept constantly aware of the troubles in the world.

Experts agree that our preoccupation with doing more things in less time is one of the most detrimental stressors of the modern era. We attempt to multi-task and feverishly try to cram as much as possible into each and every waking moment. We no longer stop to smell the flowers.

While going faster can sometimes be beneficial in the world of commerce, in the world of longevity it brings few benefits. The kind of person referred to as a 'type A' is characterised by suffering from a sort of 'hurry disease', which manifests in great impatience and dissatisfaction with oneself and with others, constant irritability, loss of temper and a great need for control. In other words, the classic workaholic.

Our fast-paced lifestyle puts enormous pressure on our lives, which also has an impact on our susceptibility to disease and ultimately leads to premature ageing. We worry too much about accumulating more and more, strive harder and harder to gain that next promotion, earn more and more money – all the while failing to ask the simple question: 'Is all this making me happy?'

Worry and Anger – The Draining Emotions

We are all basically aware that a constant state of worry or anger is physically draining and ultimately very unhealthy. These emotions have been proven to increase our risk of cancer, heart disease and stroke, although science is only just coming to understand why and how.

Are we exaggerating the significance of emotions? Well, it is actually likely that the opposite is true and that we may be under-estimating their significance. The American Institute of Stress believes that up to 90 per cent of all visits to your GP are a direct result of emotionally related disorders. A Harvard study of heart attack survivors found that feeling anger due to conflicts doubled people's chances of another heart attack. A second Harvard study identified that people who worried about their finances, social situation or health had a dramatically increased risk of developing heart disease.

Studies indicate that if you learn how to manage emotional stress, your chances of developing a life-threatening illness are almost halved. The Live-Long Code Mind Programme, by teaching you how exactly to manage stress, will kick-start your quest for a long, healthy life.

The Conscious and the Subconscious Mind

An iceberg is a good analogy to describe the connection between the conscious and the subconscious mind; there is in both a small, obvious part above the surface and a vast part below. The conscious mind is responsible for our awareness when we are awake and is what we use for thinking analytically and creating logical order. The conscious mind is responsible for cognitive learning and understanding, and utilises your intellect to come up with logical solutions for problems. It helps you to make choices based on facts and is responsible for deliberate movements of the body.

The subconscious, or unconscious, mind (these terms are inter-changeable) is the part of our mind that usually operates below any level of conscious awareness. As with the iceberg analogy, the subconscious mind is much larger than the conscious and a much more substantial and responsible part of your mind. The emotional mind is part of our subconscious, which explains why we some-times feel a certain way without really knowing why. We use our subconscious mind to store memories from the past – although not all memories are clear or easily accessible; indeed, one role of the subconscious mind is to seal off traumatic events that it is better for us to forget.

Your subconscious mind works 24 hours a day, 7 days a week; it sustains your breathing, digestion and heartbeat, grows your hair and nails, controls an enormous number of muscles to co-ordinate every single movement, and also regulates your body's temperature, water content and sugar levels. As well as all these functions, your subconscious also controls your body's self-regeneration, including producing a complete new skeleton every few years, cultivating brand new soft tissue every three months, a new liver every six weeks, eight square metres of new skin every four weeks, and a complete new stomach lining every five days! In fact, 98 per cent of the cells in your body are replaced every year. Our bodies would obviously not work as effectively and harmoniously without the involvement of the subconscious mind. It takes control of all of these automatic movements and patterns, not to mention approximately 75 per cent of daily activities, without the conscious mind needing to be involved or even aware.

Looking at the extensive duties of the subconscious mind, its power and importance become very obvious. With the right leverage and access to this power we can achieve amazing things; the subconscious mind has the potential to create profound and long-lasting changes on mental, emotional and physical levels.

Let's now focus on how to apply the subconscious mind to create long and lasting mental and physical health.

Seven-Step Live-Long Code Mind Programme

The Live-Long Code Mind Programme sets the foundation for your prolonged health by helping to create the most appropriate mental framework for longevity. This programme is supported by the Live-Long Code CD, which is available from www.immortality code.com.

It has been recognised that a number of personality traits are conducive to healthy ageing. These are self-confidence, adaptability, independence, happiness, contentment, relaxedness, openness, sociability and having a high tolerance of others. The opposing traits can therefore be considered conducive to a shorter life. The Live-Long Code exercises in this chapter are aimed at directing your subconscious mind so that you can develop a heightened sense of these personality traits.

The Live-Long Code Stress Reduction Programme

Stress is a normal and sometimes necessary part of everyday life, and can be part and parcel of striving to achieve; it is arguable that the complete absence of stress would mean the absence of truly living. However, if handled incorrectly it can be severely detrimental to your health and compromise your work towards increased longevity. It is also your reaction to stress, rather than stress itself, that is the key factor in determining how well and how long you will live, so the secret is to understand and deal properly with the stresses in your life.

Physical Excercise to Reduce Stress

Mens sana in corpore sano (a healthy mind in a healthy body) is a famous Latin quotation. Psychological stresses can be helped greatly by focusing on the physical. Indeed, remembering the fight-or-flight response, if we react to that stress physically we are doing what this natural response was intended for, which allows the body to regain homeostasis, or balance. This is why physical activity helps to clear the mind and remove the feelings associated with stress. Chapter 6 on exercise will show you how to tailor an exercise programme to support the Live-Long Code Stress Reduction Programme. For the remainder of this chapter we will focus on the mental aspect of this programme.

How to Relax

Our ability to achieve relaxation has a lot to do with the way we were brought up, the traits inherited from our parents and the environments in which we work and live. Some people feel that they need a high degree of stress in their lives and actively avoid relaxation. In the short term this can be manageable, but in the long run a person living in a constant state of stress risks burnout and illness if they don't have access to the safety valve of relaxation. The following are relaxation techniques which are all proven methods for reducing stress. You can also find these exercises on the Live-Long Code CD, which is available from www.immortalitycode.com.

Step One: Progressive Muscle Relaxation

Progressive muscle relaxation (or PMR) is a stress management technique developed by the American physician Edmund Jacobson in the early 1920s. Jacobson found that there was a correlation between muscular tension and stress, and believed that since muscular tension generally accompanies stress, it is possible to reduce stress by learning how to release muscular tension. By guiding his patients to consciously relax muscles in their body, he was able to reduce stress-associated symptoms. He found this relaxation technique to be an effective treatment for ulcers, anxiety, depression, insomnia, irritable bowel syndrome, neck and back pain, mild phobias and hypertension.

Progressive relaxation may be practised while lying on your back or sitting in a chair with your head supported. At first you may relax only partially, but with continued practice you should be able to achieve a deep relaxation in the entire body within a few minutes. Be careful though not to overly tense the neck, back, toes or feet, as this may cause muscular cramping and discomfort.

Instructions

1. Lie on your back with your eyes closed, feet slightly apart and arms slightly away from your sides with palms upwards.
2. Allow your breathing to slow down. Turn your entire attention to the breath as it moves in and out and pause for 20 seconds.
3. Tense the muscles of your feet for 5 seconds, then gently relax. Pause in the relaxed stage for 20 seconds, then repeat.
4. Tense the muscles of your calves for 5 seconds, then relax. Let the tension go. Pause for 20 seconds, then repeat.
5. Tense the muscles of your stomach for 5 seconds, then relax. Let the tension go. Pause for 20 seconds, then repeat.
6. Tense the muscles of your chest for 5 seconds, then relax for 20 seconds, then repeat.

7. Clench your fists tightly for 5 seconds, then relax. Let the tension go for 20 seconds, then repeat.
8. Flex your elbows and tense your biceps. Hold them tight for 5 seconds, then relax and straighten arms. Pause here for 20 seconds, then repeat.
9. Tense the muscles of your neck for 5 seconds. Relax. Let the tension go. Pause here for 20 seconds, then repeat.
10. Tense the muscles of your head and face for 5 seconds, then relax. Pause for 20 seconds, then repeat.

Step Two: Deep Breathing for Relaxation

Deep breathing can have a powerful influence on our health, as it promotes relaxation. Many people when they try to breathe deeply do the precise opposite: they suck in their bellies and raise their shoulders. This is actually shallow breathing or hyperventilating, and you can find yourself breathing this way when you are under stress. This fast, shallow breathing expels carbon dioxide too quickly and has many negative effects on physical and emotional health.

When our breathing is full and deep, the belly, ribcage and lower back all expand on the inhalation and retract on the exhalation. The expansion draws the diaphragm down deeper into the abdomen, and the retraction allows the diaphragm to move more fully upwards toward the heart. These downward and upward movements of the diaphragm massage the internal organs, promote blood flow and peristalsis, and pump lymph more efficiently through the lymphatic system, which is a very important part of our immune system and relies on muscular movements – including the movements of our breath – to circulate the lymph round the body.

This slow, deep breathing, combined with the rhythmical pumping of the diaphragm, helps to activate the parasympathetic nervous system – our natural relaxation response. This regulation of the nervous system has a positive impact on our overall health.

The abdomen is one of the major areas of the body that gets tight and tense when we are stressed. This exercise, performed frequently, will have a powerful influence on your overall breathing and the way in which your body deals with stress.

1. Lie down comfortably on your back, on a bed or a mat. Position yourself with your feet flat on the floor and your knees bent (pointing upward). Become aware of your breathing for a minute or two. Notice which parts of your body your breath touches.

2. Place your hands one on top of the other on your abdomen, with the centre of your lower hand touching your navel. Notice how your breathing responds. You may find that your abdomen wants to expand as you inhale and retract as you exhale. If so, allow this to happen naturally.

3. If your abdomen seems tight, massage around the outside edge of your belly button. You may notice that it begins to soften and relax.

4. If your abdomen still seems tight and does not want to move as you breathe, press down with your hands as you exhale. Then as you inhale, gradually release the tension. Try this several times. Notice how your abdomen begins to open more on inhalation.

5. As you finish, become aware of your entire abdominal area, noting any sensations of warmth, comfort and energy. Now spend a few minutes allowing these sensations to spread all over your abdomen and all the way back to your spine.

This simple exercise will have a hugely beneficial effect on your breathing, provided you do it on a regular basis. You can practise the exercise at any time of the day or night. Although it's easiest to practise lying down, you can also perform it sitting, standing or even walking. It is a good idea to practise it before you get out of bed in the morning. Over time, it will help slow down your breathing until you start to breathe that way naturally.

Step Three: Sleep

There is a lot of confusion about the importance of sleep. Some self-help books on the market promote the idea of sleeping no more than five hours a night. Some well-known historical figures survived on little sleep. However, just because they were world leaders doesn't mean that they were healthy; indeed, most of them were not. It was Napoleon Bonaparte who famously said about hours of sleep required, 'Six for the man, seven for the woman and eight for the fool.' However, Napoleon suffered from a long string of ailments, including depression, epilepsy, scabies, neurodermatitis, migraine, painful urination, chronic hepatitis and stomach cancer. He was also just 51 when he died.

Researchers from the University of Warwick and University College London have found that lack of sleep can more than double the risk of death from cardiovascular disease. Lack of sleep has also been shown to increase risk of weight gain, hypertension and type 2 diabetes, sometimes leading to mortality.

However, too much sleep can also be harmful; if you are someone who escapes stress through excessive sleeping, you should start trying not to sleep so much.

While you are sleeping your body is resting and refuelling; its building blocks of health and restoration start to work. Your blood pressure drops and your heartbeat and metabolism slow. This enables your body's cells to repair themselves and your body to create new cells in every one of its systems. Poor sleep weakens immune function and reduces the number of killer cells that combat germs and cells that divide too rapidly, as well as cancer cells. Studies have shown that chronic sleep deprivation also contributes to gastrointestinal problems, heart disease and a host of other medical conditions.

You know you are getting a good quality of sleep when you wake refreshed in the morning. If you are not waking refreshed, then you either are not getting enough sleep or your sleep quality is poor. Waking frequently during the night to go to the bathroom, or vivid dreams that disturb your sleep, obviously affects your sleep quality.

You should ensure that your bedroom is conducive to sleep. Remove all the clutter and make sure that your bed is comfortable. Make sure that you have comfortable, clean sheets. It is also a good idea not to overstimulate your brain before attempting to fall asleep. This means switching off the TV at least 20 minutes before retiring. If you are going to read in bed, make sure you give yourself some time to wind down after you finish reading.

As part of the Live-Long Code Programme you will learn to avoid caffeinated beverages. If you do need to have a drink before bed, consider a soothing mug of camomile tea, which is conducive to sleep. Avoid having too much to drink before bedtime, however, or your sleep may be interrupted by the need to go to the bathroom.

The Eastern system of chi kung takes the importance of sleep very seriously and uses exercise to enhance sleep. If you have problems sleeping, practise the following exercise, which is particularly effective. It should be performed sitting on your bed, with pillows at your back to fall onto as you drift into sleep.

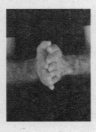

1. Clap your hands and rub them together to draw heat from your heart.

2. Massage your lower back in the kidney area (known as mingmen or Gate of Vitality) 36 times.

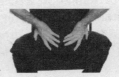

3. Place both hands over your mingmen area and take three breaths, imagining sending qi (energy) from your hands into your kidneys.

4. Repeat two or three times.

5. Place your right ankle on your left knee and your right hand on your navel. Now with your left hand gently massage the sole of the right foot until you start to fall asleep.

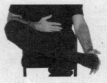

Many people have difficulty sleeping when they are stressed. Others, perhaps by choice, don't allow themselves enough sleep and feel more stressed in daily life due to tiredness. A restful night and enough sleep, though, are key ingredients in helping to deal with life's daily stresses. If you cannot actually avoid stress, making sure that you get a good night's sleep is one of the most important things you can to do to help you deal with that stress.

Step Four: Become Fluent in the Language of Immortality

Why are some people optimistic and others pessimistic? There are a number of factors, including the society in which we live, the way our parents spoke to us and the manner in which we were educated. There are even genetic traits that contribute to our personal level of optimism. However, ultimately optimism is a trait that can be learned; the key to this is to understand the language we use and, in particular, the internal language we direct at ourselves. You might think that this self-dialogue is built-in, but it isn't; many of us have got into the habit of speaking very harshly towards ourselves. We can all learn to develop a self-dialogue that is conducive to positivity, high performance, optimism and, ultimately, greater happiness. And we can gain fluency at any age.

The Voices in Your Head

For all of us there is a constant conversation going on in our heads which affects every aspect of our lives.

Every day we have choices to make that affect the course of our lives. But on a more subtle level, we are actually making choices in every moment, by choosing the thoughts that we have. Those choices, to a great degree, will determine how our lives unfold. Most people may think that thoughts 'just happen' and that they are not responsible for those thoughts. But whether we are aware of it or not, we create our own thoughts and they manifest in the language that we use.

Mind/body medicine reveals that our mental state, or frame of mind, can alter the way our bodies feel, which in turn has an impact on overall health. We can empower ourselves to change the state of our health and the quality of our life by changing our thinking from negative to positive, moment by moment.

From the moment we wake in the morning we engage in a constant self-dialogue. From the work I do with my clients I have found that most people with anxiety, depression, low self-esteem and other psychological problems almost always have one particular trait in common: they constantly dialogue with themselves in a very harsh manner. Imagine having someone who walked around with you every day telling you that you are no good and that you always do things wrong. Well, unfortunately for many people this is precisely what happens on a constant basis – except that the 'person' or the voice accompanying them is in fact their own. The problem for many of us is that we aren't fully aware of the impact this dialogue has on our lives and our health, but if we change our thoughts for the positive we automatically improve the quality of our lives immediately, and in a very substantial way.

In order to understand how we think, we need to look at this self-dialogue. By becoming aware of the words and phrases you are using, the tone of voice and the intention behind those words, you will learn to understand the 'programming code' of your brain. It is these words that are controlling your mind and it is only by altering these words that you will reprogramme your mind for longevity.

Imagine that you are the coach of a kids' sports team. Your task is to look after the team and boost the confidence of all the players. Some of the children are nervous and afraid of making mistakes that might let the rest of the team down. One of the children on your team misses what should be an almost certain score and you notice that their head goes down and they start to play with an obvious lack of self-belief.

Close your eyes and imagine what language you would use towards the player to boost their confidence and get them back in the game, performing to the best of their ability. Notice the tone of your voice and the positive intention behind your words.

Now let's take a different perspective. I want you to imagine that *you* are a player on a team. You have been given a really easy scoring opportunity and instead of putting your team in the lead you completely miss-hit the ball and fall over.

Close your eyes and notice the things you say to yourself. Notice the tone and the intention of your words. Notice how you feel. Do you imagine that the other players are cursing you or that some of the opposition or the people on the sideline are laughing at you? How are the words different from the way you would talk to the child on the team you are trying to help? Is it harsh where the other was comforting?

The point here is that we do not generally allow other people to talk to us as harshly as we talk to ourselves. Yet our self-dialogue rules our lives. So if you learn to change this dialogue, you can literally change the course of your life.

Successful sportspeople all have a highly developed positive self-dialogue when it comes to their own performance. For some athletes this is so powerful that they cannot even contemplate any sort of failure, so when defeat finally comes to their door they are ill-prepared to deal with it. In this context some great sportsmen, like Prince Naseem Hamed and even the formidable Mike Tyson, faded away fairly quickly once the spell of their invincibility had been broken. This is why the true sporting legends are the ones who can taste defeat and still come back better; they have the mental strength to take a defeat and somehow internalise it with a positive slant so that they can come back stronger than before. Muhammad Ali is generally considered to be one of the greatest mental athletes of all time, and he lost and regained the world heavyweight boxing title a record three times.

You might think of another sporting great like John McEnroe and perhaps contend that some of his rantings and tantrums weren't particularly positive. But if we take a closer look at McEnroe we see a huge sense of belief in his own ability, which extended to his ability to see better than the umpires and court officials. McEnroe's anger and frustration were generally directed towards 'morons' – other people – and very rarely towards himself.

Now, without being judgemental I want you to observe your own everyday inner self-dialogue. Do you recognise any of the following types of self-dialogue statements? 'There you go again – you do this all the time.' 'Why do you always do that?' 'Why am I so stupid?' 'You stupid ass.' 'Oh no, I wish I could just stay in bed.' 'I'm such a fool.' You might be able to think of some harsher examples.

The leading psychologist Shad Helmstetter has estimated that 77 per cent of all self-dialogue is negative and counterproductive. Whether you realise it or not, what you are putting into your brain in the form of this self-dialogue is what you will get back out. It affects every aspect of our lives, including our behaviour, our relationships, our work and, ultimately, our sense of well-being. Your subconscious works hard to manifest whatever you tell it, so by programming your mind with words and intentions you are implementing what is known as the law of self-fulfilling prophesy.

When faced with adversity it is understandable that you may talk to yourself negatively, but it is actually at these times that negative self-dialogue is particularly unhelpful. It is important to remember that the intention behind this self-dialogue is actually positive – your harsh words are meant to discourage yourself from making mistakes and to encourage you to do things better. But unless your self-dialogue is conducted in a way that is constructive and positive, it almost always will not benefit you at all.

Your self-dialogue ultimately provides the instructions and directions for your subconscious mind. Therefore, every time you make a negative statement about yourself or your sense of health or well being, you are directing your subconscious mind to make you become the person you've described.

The Vocabulary of Immortality

In our culture in the UK and Ireland, success is sometimes resented and failure celebrated. Our brothers and sisters in the United States do not seem to have the same stifling problem. How often when you are asked, 'How are you doing?' do you respond 'Not too bad' or 'It could be worse'? When you think about it, these phrases actually say that you are not doing good, which delivers a message to your subconscious to that effect. What's wrong with using words like 'outstanding' and 'fantastic' to describe how you are? If you use negative language it trains your subconscious not to *expect* to have a great day. And as we know, what our subconscious expects is generally what we get. It is therefore important that from now on you get used to phrasing things in the most positive manner possible. And, get this, phrase things even more positively when things aren't totally fantastic – just yet.

We want to phrase things in the most positive way possible in order to train our subconscious to manifest positive outcomes. Take a moment right now to write down some of the words and phrases that you have used in the past that could have made you feel bad. At the time you may not have realised that this was going to be the effect, but now you know better. Words like 'depressed', 'angry', 'in pain', 'anxious'. When you have compiled a full list of these frequently used words, think of some alternative words and phrases to change the emotional intensity. For example, 'depressed' could change to 'on the way back', 'angry' to 'irritated', 'pain' could be 'discomfort'. Whenever you find yourself using a word or phase that has strong negative intent, add it to your list and find an alternative, more positive word or phrase. Here are some ideas to get you started.

Negative Word	Changes To
Acute	Temporary
Aching	Niggling
Annoyed	Irked
Afraid	Uncomfortable
Alone	Waiting for a friend
Anxious	Restless
Chronic	Frequent
Disturbed	Moved
Exhausted	Gathering energy
Failed	Moving towards success
Frightened	Challenged
Helpless	Welcoming support
Hopeless	Needing encouragement

Hurting	Uncomfortable
Lonely	Bored
Nervous	Expectant
Not too bad	Fantastic
Overwhelmed	In demand
Out of control	Making changes
Painful	Uncomfortable
Scared	Eager
Sick	Recovering
Stressed	Energised
Traumatised	Moved to action
Useless	Not required

Step Five: Meditation

Without a doubt, meditation is one of the most effective ways to improve our response to stress. Meditation is practised by thousands of people around the world on a daily basis. However, many people mistakenly believe that meditation is too complex and too difficult to do. In fact, meditation, like many things, simply is a skill that takes a bit of learning and which improves with practice.

Meditation is a key component of the Live-Long Code. You should integrate it into your life and use it often. As you develop your meditation skills, you may well find that your practice improves your clarity of thought and your decision-making ability and generally helps you to organise your thoughts. As a result you will be better able to handle stress and the daily disruptions of society.

How Meditation Works

Meditation is easy, but like all skills you need to learn how to do it. The first surprise often comes when you realise just how undisciplined your mind really is and how it sometimes simply refuses to abide by your will. As a test, just try to count your breath for five minutes without thinking about anything else. One of the objectives of meditation is to train your mind to focus on what you want it to. As part of this aim you will, with practice, learn to empty your mind and think of nothing.

When you learn to empty your mind you will free yourself from the stresses of daily life that prevent your mind from resting, sometimes even when you are asleep.

How Meditation Can Benefit You Physically

Meditation produces a deep state of physiological relaxation, lowers the metabolic rate (the rate at which we expend energy) and decreases heart and respiration rates. Our parasympathetic nervous system is stimulated, which improves digestion and causes an overall relaxation response. This counteracts the fight-or-flight response associated with stress and anxiety.

This lower metabolism and heart rate, together with the lower oxygen requirement, causes a decrease in carbon dioxide produced and lowers the concentration in the blood of lactic acid, which at high levels is associated with anxiety and stress. Studies into this have shown that blood lactic acid levels in people who meditate are only a quarter of those of the average person who doesn't meditate. We still have a great deal to learn about meditation, but the more research that is conducted, the more we are learning about the considerable benefits of this practice.

Preparing Your Mind for Meditation

This exercise is a powerful way to prepare yourself for meditation that will turbo-charge you towards a powerfully positive, resourceful state and will also be the perfect preparation for the meditation you will enjoy later as part of the Live-Long Code Mind Programme.

Reprogramme Your Mind for Living Longer

Stage One – Thought Awareness

Find a place where you can relax completely. Sit comfortably on a chair or lie on a bed. Allowing your body to relax, close your eyes and simply observe the ebb and flow of your thoughts for five minutes. Remember the progression of these thoughts. When you begin this exercise you are likely to notice that your thoughts relate to matters of everyday life; home- or work-related matters or worries may rush in on you. Your thoughts may also seem quite haphazard and somewhat chaotic. At this stage you should simply maintain the position of a silent observer, independently watching the flow of these thoughts. Depending on your state of mind this exercise will be difficult or easy. When difficulties occur, try to maintain your train of thought and observe attentively.

Start by practising this exercise twice a day; begin with five minutes and then extend the duration by one minute each time you perform it until you are observing your thoughts for 10 minutes. Write down a brief note on your train of thought.

In the beginning you are likely to be besieged by thoughts, but as you practise, your thoughts will quickly become less indiscriminate. When you have mastered this exercise your thoughts will be slow, ordered and easily remembered. It is when you have achieved this that you are ready to move to the next stage – thought control.

Stage Two – Thought Control: Empowering a Positive Self-Dialogue

At this stage of the exercise you are going to take more conscious control of your thoughts, refusing to allow any negative self-dialogue to linger in your thoughts. If any negative thought or discouraging sentiment, such as 'Why do you make silly mistakes?', pops into your head, acknowledge the intent of the message, which in this case is that you want to perform the activity better, and then immediately remove the negative statement from your mind.

Just imagine gathering the negative thought and literally cleaning it out of your mind. Visualise yourself wiping it off a whiteboard and say 'ERASE' in your head as you do so. Then replace the thought with a more positive equivalent phrase, such as 'I'm learning to improve'.

If you find yourself slipping up, avoid self-criticism, as this simply exacerbates the issue. Move on and practise this part of the exercise until you can comfortably follow your thoughts for 10 minutes without allowing any negative thoughts to linger.

Stage Three – Thought Mastery: The Seven-Day Live-Long Code Mental Reprogramme

The final part of this exercise has far-reaching and empowering benefits. During this stage you will learn to retain a consistent state of mental positivity that will have a direct impact on your psychology and consequently on your entire life. For seven consecutive days you will refuse to dwell on any negative self-dialogue. This is to be practised throughout your day. By this stage you will have developed the thought awareness to monitor your thoughts and the skills to control your thoughts. Now you will reject all negative thoughts immediately and retain that constant mental state of positivity over a prolonged period of time. Each thought must be reframed and transformed from a negative thought to become a positive thought, or else just rejected completely.

When you notice the beginning of any negative self-dialogue, immediately use the 'ERASE' method from Step Two. For these seven days you will train your mind to focus on positive solutions. As soon as you are confronted with a mental or physical challenge, immediately focus your intention on what you want the solution to be.

If you falter and find yourself lingering on negative self-dialogue for any length of time, just accept that you need to continue to work on this exercise and launch the Seven-Day Live-Long Code Mental Reprogramme from the beginning. Consistency is the key component of this exercise and therefore it is important to begin again at day one if you do slip up. This will ensure that by the end of the seven days, your mind is repatterned to consistently move towards positive self-dialogue, having perfected the retention of a constant state of mental assuredness.

Give yourself plenty of time to master this exercise. Persist with it; the rewards are enormous and it will have a profoundly positive impact on you and your life. When you have completed this stage of the exercise you are ready to practise meditation, and your skills will continue to develop the more you practise.

How to Meditate

We know that meditation is probably one of the most effective and efficient methods of relaxation. By now you will have practised many of the skills required for mediation by performing the previous exercises in this chapter. The key to meditation for relaxation is to focus on one relaxing thought for a sustained period of time. This calms your mind and gives your body time to relax and recuperate and clear away toxic thoughts that may have built up through stress and mental activity.

The essence of meditation is to quieten your thoughts by focusing completely on just one thing. Hypnotic trance is somewhat similar, although this is often more of a passive experience. Meditation is an active process that seeks to exclude outside thoughts by concentrating your full mental focus on the meditation subject. Meditation should be performed in a position that you can comfortably sustain for a period of time – ideally 20 minutes or so. Sitting in a comfortable chair or lying on a bed can be effective; in certain circumstances you can even meditate while walking.

The following are the key elements to meditation.

- **Set aside time to meditate.**
  Make available at least a little time every day to meditate. The effects of meditation are far more significant when you practise it regularly and consistently than if your practice is occasional.

  You can meditate at any time of day, but I think morning meditation is an ideal start to the day. You may also like to meditate at the end of the day, as it is good practice to clear your mind before going to sleep. If you have a stressful job you may prefer to find sanctuary in meditation in the middle of a busy day. Generally, however, it is easier to meditate in the morning, before the day's events tire your body out and stimulate your mind too much.

- **Meditate in a quiet, relaxing place.**
  When you're starting your practice of meditation, it's important to avoid distractions. Switch off your TV, phone, radio and anything else that may cause distraction. If you do want to meditate to music, use sounds that are calm, repetitive and gentle and do not contain vocals. You can also meditate outside but, again, make sure that the location is peaceful.

- **Find a comfortable posture.**
  It's important to feel physically relaxed when meditating, as any discomfort can cause distraction. You do not have to twist your limbs into the lotus position or adopt any unusual postures, but it is important while sitting to keep your back straight, as this will help with breathing later on.

  Any position in which you're relaxed but your back is straight is good. You can practise meditation lying down, but be aware that the deep sense of relaxation you achieve may cause you to fall asleep.

  Begin each exercise by taking in a deep breath and gently letting it out. As you breathe, allow yourself to start to relax. When you've completed the exercise, slowly and gently re-activate yourself by breathing a little more deeply, wiggling your fingers and toes, and opening your eyes when you feel ready.

- **Unfocus your eyes.**
  Allow your eyes to half close without focusing on anything. If this is challenging for you, close your eyes or else find something steady to focus on, such as a small candle flame. Breathe deeply and slowly from your abdomen. You should feel your stomach rise and fall while your chest stays relatively still. We have looked at abdominal breathing, and you may perform this by inhaling for a count of three and exhaling for a count of six, and repeating. This expels all used air from your lungs and more completely oxygenates your blood, helping to lower heart rate and blood pressure.

- **Relax the muscles in your body.**
  Take your time to relax. Clench your fists together and pull your forearms tightly up against your upper arms. While keeping those muscles tense, next tense all the muscles in your legs. Then clench your jaws and shut your eyes tight. Now, holding everything tense, take a deep breath and hold it for five seconds. Then breathe out and let all of your muscles go at once. Feel yourself letting go of all your tension. Enjoy that feeling of relaxation as your muscles let go more and more.

- **Focus your attention.**
  If your mind wants to wander, moving from thought to thought, gently bring your focus back to a single point until it rests there naturally. The goal is to allow the 'chattering' in your mind to gradually fade away.

  It's a good idea to allow your attention to move to your breath. Listen to it, follow it, without making any comments or judgements about it, such as 'It seems short . . . or perhaps I'm getting a cold?' To overcome verbal chatter you may find it useful to count breaths. Count your breaths from one to ten and then start again at one.

  To thwart images that try to intrude into your thoughts, visualise a place that calms you. It can be a real place you know, or an imaginary one. You could imagine descending a staircase that leads to a tranquil and relaxing place.

- **Quieten your mind.**
  Once you've trained your mind to focus on just one thing at a time, you can practise the next step, which is to focus on nothing at all. Essentially this means 'clearing' your mind. After spending a while focusing on a single point, such as your breath, as described in the previous steps, you can allow it to drift away, or observe it impartially as you let it come and go, again without labelling it or making internal comments. Take the same approach to any thoughts that return to your mind, until you achieve silence.

- **You can take relaxation practice anywhere.**
  With practise, you will become more skilled at relaxing while
  awake, anywhere you need to, at will. You will be able to do it
  while walking, or while sitting in class or at work.

Guided Meditation

Guided meditation is a technique in which the person is led
through the meditative process by a soothing voice that helps
the individual to achieve a state of peacefulness and clarity. In
many cases, hypnotic techniques such as the use of repetitive
phrases can be helpful in deepening the meditative state. The
calming voice may also include language that helps to conjure
up images that promote the sense of inner calm that comes with
meditation.

Guided meditation is helpful for people who are just beginning
their meditative practice. The Immortality Code CD includes a
powerful guided meditation and is available from www.immortality
code.com. You can have someone read a guided meditation script
to you, or record your own and play it back to yourself. If you don't
like recording and hearing your own voice you can ask a friend to
record it for you. Remember, it should be read slowly and in a soft
pitch and tone.

The idea is that you allow your conscious mind to switch off
while following the words that are being spoken on a subconscious
level. What many people like about guided meditation is that they
can effortlessly achieve a deep state of relaxation or even sleep while
still retaining subconscious awareness.

Guided Meditation Script

This is a very brief guided meditation that encourages self-healing.
It will give you a feel for how guided meditation works.

> Begin by sitting comfortably but with your back supported, and
> allow your body to relax. Your feet are touching the ground, with

your arms relaxed in your lap. Now notice your breathing. Notice how steady and relaxed it is. Notice how steady it is – first in . . . then out. As you breathe in, visualise clean, white energy filling your lungs. Then, as you breathe out, feel any toxins or stress exit your body in a grey mist.

Breathe in the white, and breathe out the grey, keeping that same slow but steady beat. Focus on the increasing feeling of relaxation for 10 deep inhalations and 10 full exhalations. Notice the energy that is in your body and notice the sensations of warmth and comfort that begin to permeate each cell in your body. Notice the sensations of the energy around you on the surface of your skin. As you relax deeper, feel the external energies and internal energies blend together.

Now visualise warm, soothing energy shining down from above your head. Bring this shining, glowing energy down through the top of your head and feel it melting like warm oil, down into your body. Feel it melt relaxation down the front of your face, your neck, your shoulders and down into your arms. Feel this energy melting through every cell and fibre in your body, down your chest, into your abdomen, down your hips and all the way down your legs to your toes.

Notice that your whole body is filled with healing light and energy, and observe that your legs and your body feel lighter. Allow this healing energy to completely fill your physical space as you bask in a deep sense of relaxation. You may want to smile as you feel a beautiful, warm, glowing sensation all over. Let go even farther, going deeper and deeper. Sit in the golden light, and focus on your slow, occasional breathing. Keep focusing for as long as you want the meditation to continue, then when you want to finish take a breath in and slowly start to wiggle your fingers and toes. Gradually lift and stretch your arms and, when you feel ready, increase the movements and then slowly open your eyes, feeling bright and alert and feeling great!

The Immortality Code CD contains a more extensive guided meditation than this one, which incorporates music and numerous supporting techniques. When you begin practising your guided meditation regularly, you will feel more relaxed and find that you can cope with stress more easily. This in turn enhances your immunity and general sense of well being. When you consider how much time you have spent in the past, worrying and rushing, it seems only fair that you now enjoy greater and deeper relaxation. Guided meditation is an effective way to help you achieve this.

Creating Your Life Vision

Muhammad Ali, known the world over as 'The Greatest', is generally accepted as the most supreme mental athlete in living memory. Ali won most of his fights long before he ever set foot in the ring. In preparation for a fight, how many times would you guess Muhammad Ali contemplated the ways in which he might lose a fight? The answer of course is that he would never contemplate losing a fight! He convinced his subconscious mind that he was invincible by repeatedly focusing his attention only on the ways in which he would win. He was so good at this that not only did he train his subconscious mind for victory, but he also trained his opponent's subconscious mind for defeat. He did this by writing and reciting poetry describing how and when in the fight he would beat his victim. Most of his opponents listened and played their role to bring these words to life in the ring. Remember that the nickname 'The Greatest' was after all given to Ali by the great man himself. He even trained you and me! Muhammad Ali was brilliant at developing a clear, positive vision of success. This vision was so clear that making it happen eventually became not much more than a formality.

Now ask yourself this question: What do I want in relation to prolonging my life and retaining good health? Many people would answer this question by saying that they do not want a particular illness or health problem. But remember that you always get more of what you focus on. So just as Muhammad Ali would only focus on winning a fight, we must redirect our focus and consequently our subconscious mind on our goal – which is full health rather than 'no illness'. By being clear about the vision of full health as opposed to the absence of illness, we are directing ourselves to move towards that vision. The more clearly and vividly we create that vision of health, the more accurately we train our subconscious mind to deliver it to our bodies.

So let's create a solid vision of your healthy future by developing a Well-Formed Outcome.

Step Six: Creating a Well-Formed Outcome

Clear objectives make us focus our attention. You wouldn't go to the ticket office of a train station and ask for a ticket without telling the cashier where you wanted to go. Similarly, not knowing precisely what you want in terms of your healthy longevity can lead to a lack of clarity in what you want to achieve, and make you less likely to be prepared for success. There is an old saying in Chinese medicine: 'Wherever the mind goes, the body will follow.' This exercise steers your mind towards prolonged health and longevity, to the benefit of your body.

This technique was developed by the genius mind of Dr Richard Bandler, the founder of neurolinguistic programming (NLP), and will enable you to consciously train and direct your subconscious mind towards successful and healthy longevity.

1. State your life and future health and longevity goals in the positive. This means that rather than stating something like 'I don't want to have a walking stick' you would say 'I want my walking to be balanced and strong'.

_____

_____

_____

_____

_____

In a famous study, two rowing teams of similar ability repeatedly raced against each other, taking turns at repeating two different mantras: 'We will win' and 'We will not lose'. Time and again the team that recited 'We will win' would come out as the victor, even though both teams took random turns at using both phrases.

The subconscious mind, curiously, deletes words like 'not' and so will often direct you in the opposite direction to the one you really want to go. As an example, I want you NOT to think of a pig giraffe. What picture did you create in your mind? You understand the point.

Now choose your outcome – and don't have any half measures. Make it a powerful and positive goal that fully captures the full vision of your future.

2. Next I want you to be more specific about the outcome you want. In what way precisely do you want to live your life? How will your good health manifest itself? State precisely, in a POSITIVE way, how you want to be living your life. Detail the healthy way in which you want to live as you get older. For example, detail beginning a new career five years from now. Or, having learned a new language, you travel to the country where it's spoken in your eighty-fifth year. Or celebrating your hundredth birthday party with friends and family at your favourite destination.

_____

_____

_____

3. Now I want you to answer the 'W' questions:

• What is the current stage you are at in relation to this objective?

_____

• When do you want this to happen?

_____

• Where do you want this to take place?

_____

• Who are the people who will benefit from this outcome?

_____

• What will achieving this outcome do for you?

_____

• What will you do with your life after you have achieved this outcome?

_____

4. How will you verify that it has happened? Answer the following questions relating to your senses.

• What will you hear when you achieve it?

_____

• What will you hear from your friends, family and relatives?

_____

• What will you see when you achieve it? For example, smiles, tears of joy, your improved appearance in the mirror, healthy complexion.

_____

• What will you feel when you achieve it? For example, physical sensations of joy, love, happiness, excitement, pride, strength, relief.

_____

• What will you smell or taste? Perhaps you will taste celebratory champagne.

_____

5. Will you lose anything if you achieve this outcome? We will come back to this topic again later in the chapter. But think: what secondary gains does your illness give you that you will have to give up in order to achieve your chosen outcome? For example, bad habits, free time, attention, care from family and friends, control, comfort.

_____

6. How will your life change after you achieve the Well-Formed Outcome?

_____

8. How will you start taking action to get your Well-Formed Outcome now? For example, you will read and implement this book. What else will you do?

_____

Step Seven: Positive Visualisation

When we think, we do so in words and in pictures. We have looked at the importance of maintaining a positive self-dialogue and positive vocabulary even in everyday communication. Equally important is to have a positive self-image that you move towards with ever-increasing certainty. The following exercise trains your brain to envisage a complete sense of health and vitality. Just as an athlete visualises sporting success and then frequently goes on to achieve it, you too will create a vision of yourself with a full sense of vitality and you will use this vision as your immediate physical and health goal. Perform this exercise every day.

Programming Your Self-Image for Health and Longevity

Sit comfortably on a chair. Allow your eyes to close as your body starts to relax. With each breath feel your body relax more deeply. Now imagine yourself, looking completely healthy and invigorated, standing right in front of you. This is your True Self. Take some time to notice the characteristics of your True Self. Notice the way you stand confidently, breathe, smile and move. Notice the way the true healthy you interacts with others.

Now, step inside your True Self. See what you can see through bright, healthy eyes. Hear through the ears of your True Self. Breathe comfortably and in a relaxed way as your True Self and sense just how good it feels to be strong and healthy.

Finish the programming session by allowing some time to visualise just how great your life will be as you live it as your True Self.

Age-Proofing Your Brain

Can you exercise your brain in such a way as to age-proof it? This is the question that drives an industry of brain-training software and gadgets. The short answer is that because our brain changes in response to experience and learning, it can also be trained and protected by brain exercises. This is the premise of the various kinds of cognitive rehabilitation exercises in existence that are used for people who have experienced a stroke.

One brain trainer, developed by Posit Science (www.positscience.com), has gone through numerous clinical trials. Their training programme requires an initially fairly significant, short-term time commitment – about an hour a day for a month. The programme was developed by University of California-San Francisco neuroscientist Michael Merzenich. Dr Merzenich's hypothesis is that as the brain gets older it has more difficulty filtering out distractions. Consequently, information doesn't get into the brain as efficiently. The Posit program helps you make fine distinctions with your ears, and improves your auditory processing. Once your brain has been trained to hear more clearly, you will also remember more clearly. In a trial involving nearly 600 participants at the Mayo Clinic and the University of Southern California, this is exactly what happened: participants who went through the Posit protocol tested 10 years younger on their memory tests.

A more recent study, by Dr Gary Small of the University of California in Los Angeles (UCLA), has shown that surfing the web is good for age-proofing the brain. Researchers found that both reading and searching for material on the internet increased activity in several parts of the brain, including those that control language, reading, memory and visual abilities.

Some functions of the brain, such as language skills and long-term memory, can continue to sharpen as you get older provided that you stay mentally active. The brain can be trained just as the muscles in your body can. If you want your brain to operate optimally, you need to use and exercise it regularly.

The best advice if you want to retain a youthful brain is to use and challenge it every day. Get into the habit of doing brain-challenging activities as often as possible. Learning a new language also can help, and research suggests that eating certain foods and avoiding other foods can help to age-proof the brain. A 2008 British study found that eating blueberries can enhance memory and learning. Of course nutrition affects both your mind and body; therefore we are going to optimise your diet for both physical and mental longevity.

You will have realised that it is practically impossible to completely avoid or escape stress. We have also looked at how stress is a necessary part of life and that it can be beneficial – provided you know how to deal with it in the correct way.

Stress management with the methods covered in this chapter, building to a daily routine of meditation, is a key element of the Live-Long Code. A successful stress management programme will also include elements from the rest of the Live-Long Code Programme, including exercise, proper nutrition and supplements as well as detoxification.

Summary

- You have learned some powerful new ways to run your own brain. When you consistently practise these exercises, you will alter the software in your head and manifest powerful benefits and changes to the way you feel very quickly. By embracing these techniques, you will not only benefit your health, but also significantly enhance the quality of your life and the lives of the people around you.

- Indulge yourself in consistent mental positivity. Continue to work through this book, but also spend time working on the mind-programming exercises in this chapter. You have already been called upon to perform exercises that will have created the mental foundation for long-lasting health and longevity.

- Some of the exercises you need only perform once. For example, you only write your health recovery story once and produce one Well-Formed Outcome. Other techniques, such as the Three Steps to Reprogramme Your Mind exercise, you will practise for the next couple of weeks and come back to them later as and when you wish.

- Incorporating 20 minutes of meditation into your daily routine is one of the most effective ways to manage stress. Anybody who meditates for any length of time will sometimes reach a plateau. The key is to have the persistence and discipline to continue and make new breakthroughs. Excellent meditation requires good preparation and practice.

- The Immortality Code CD is available from www.immortalitycode. com; the CD supports this chapter and guides you through many of the techniques. Use it to help implement an ongoing Mind Programme for Immortality.

Perhaps one of the most important lessons of this chapter is that YOU are responsible for the way your mind operates. From now on it's your choice. YOU are in control.

With your mind primed for immortality, next we must turn to a scientifically proven way to dramatically extend your healthy lifespan – by as much as 20 years. It's time to look at your nutrition and the foods of immortality.

CHAPTER FOUR

The Live-Long Code
Nutrition Plan

The food that you eat provides the essential energy that your body needs to live. The objective of the Live-Long Code Nutrition Plan is not weight loss, although if you are overweight a positive side effect of the eating plan is that you are likely to lose weight rapidly. The Live-Long Diet involves a lifestyle approach to nutrition that will significantly enhance your prospects of longevity. To succeed with the plan it helps to have a full understanding of what it is and why it works.

The Live-Long Code Nutrition Plan consists of three elements:

1. Calorie restriction.
2. Optimum nutrition.
3. Proven supplementation.

Now let's look at each of these components in depth.

Calorie Restriction

There is a proven elixir of youth that nearly all scientists agree can turn back or at least slow the ageing process, as well as improving quality of life as you age. This elixir is known as calorie restriction.

Our tendency to overindulge with food is a survival instinct that for the most part, in modern Western society, is redundant. In our earlier evolution, when it wasn't certain where our next meal was going to come from, it served a purpose to overindulge when food was available. This provided stores of energy that would hopefully tide us over until our next meal. But for most of us in the modern world, with access to our next meal no longer in doubt, this instinct to eat more than is necessary needs to be held in check.

Calorie restriction is a proven method to reverse the ageing process. In many controlled laboratory studies, restricting calorie intake has always resulted in the test animals living a longer and more functional life with less chronic disease. Studies on rats have shown an incredible increase in lifespan, from an average of 101 days to 197 days. Human studies have tried to find out why the Okinawans of Japan have more than four times the centenarians of other Japanese. From a nutritional perspective, the Okinawans eat three times more vegetables, twice as much fish and one-third fewer calories than in the standard Japanese diet. It will take many more years of scientific research to fully understand the mechanism of how calorie restriction works within the human body. There is, however, no doubt that it works.

Calorie Restriction Is Not Malnourishment

Calorie restriction should not be thought of as malnutrition or extended fasting. As these practices can create nutritional deficiencies, they can actually accelerate the ageing process. By contrast, when calorie restriction is properly performed it provides the body with all the nutrients it needs but does not overburden your system. When you eat more food than is required, your body has to work harder to digest it, and if that energy is not utilised your body stores what you don't need in the form of fat. If you restrict your food intake to what is required to maintain a healthy and active lifestyle, your body regulates its metabolic rate to conserve the limited amount of energy it receives. This is your body's innate mechanism for self-preservation.

When we eat we cannot help but produce free radicals as a by-product. This results in oxidation. Therefore, overeating leads to an increased oxidation level, increased fat storage and an excessive insulin load and sugar imbalance. With less calorie intake and less food for your body to digest, there is less oxidative damage and consequently less ageing. Also, the slowing down of your organ system gives your internal organs more rest and prolongs their lifespan. Healthy organs again mean longer life.

Scientists do not yet fully understand why calorific restriction has such powerful anti-ageing effects, but a few of the theories are as follows:

1. That ageing is caused by a build-up of oxidative damage. It has been established that animals placed on a restricted calorie diet have less of this type of damage. Therefore, the hypothesis is that calorie restriction slows metabolism and thus slows oxidation, creating less cellular damage (Koubova and Guarente, 2003).

2. An accumulation of damaged proteins in the body may also be a cause of ageing. Calorie restriction seems to speed up the protein turnover rate and therefore may hinder the build-up of damaged proteins. This may happen due to the body breaking down protein when it has run short of fat to burn (Koubova, 2003).

3. Ageing is associated with an increased rate of cellular death. Calorie restriction may work by increasing the long-term survival rate of irreplaceable cells. A key regulator of cell defenses in response to stress is the enzyme SIRT1. When one is engaged in caloric restriction, SIRT1 is released in many of the body's tissues and cell survival is increased (Cohen et al., 2004).

If calorie restriction was carried to the extreme it would be damaging and actually accelerate ageing. The body requires food to generate energy. During extreme fasting, malnutrition or starvation, the body breaks down muscles and organ structures for energy; this is very destructive and compromises health and lifespan.

Calorie Restriction	*Anorexia*
Motivation is a long healthy life	Motivation is to be in control by starving oneself
Seek support from physicians to ensure meeting nutritional needs	Hide condition from physicians and others
Come in all shapes and sizes	Drastically underweight
Concerned with achieving optimal nutrition with as few calories as possible	Concerned with consuming as few calories as possible or not eating; have no concern for nutrition
Mind not preoccupied with food	Mind preoccupied by eating disorder

The Benefits Of Calorie Restriction

Calorific restriction has the folowing benefits: lowered systolic blood pressure, improved immune system function, improved thyroid function, improved cardiovascular health, reduced risk of autoimmune disease, and reduced incidence of lymphoma, kidney disease and certain cancers.

In fact, calorie restriction has been proven to reduce the incidence of nearly all the diseases we associate with ageing:

- Cancer.
- Heart disease.
- Diabetes.
- Osteoporosis.
- Autoimmune disorders.
- Neurological decline.
- Alzheimer's disease.
- Parkinson's disease.

The physiological benefits of calorie restriction are many and include:

- Increased lifespan.
- Improved learning ability (sharper mind).
- Increased neurotransmitter receptors (clearer mind).
- Reduced fat accumulation (better body contour).
- Decreased insulin level (better sugar control).
- Reduced incidence of cancer (less oxidative damage).
- Reduced rate of heart disease (less stress on the cardiovascular system).
- Reduction in loss of bone mass (less osteoporosis).

Do you need to be on a calorie-restricted programme? Calorie restriction is not for everyone. Women who are pregnant should not follow a calorie-restrictive diet as it could possibly contribute to premature birth or low birth weight. Children and teenagers, who are still growing, should of course eat sensibly, but it would not be recommended for them to follow a calorie programme.

Let's take a closer look at how to determine if you would benefit from a calorie-restriction programme. This is largely dictated by body weight. There are two kinds of weight measures used to determine if you are overweight or underweight:

1. Ideal body weight.
2. Live-Long Code target weight.

Your ideal body weight is a statistical average that assumes that you are an average person in your mid-twenties. The important thing to remember is that you are unique and that this ideal body weight is just a statistical tool used to give general guidance. It does not take into consideration build or any medical conditions. As such we cannot simply go by ideal body weight as a measurement, but should only use it as a general and basic guideline.

The Live-Long Code

Live-Long Code Target Weight

Your Live-Long Code target weight is the goal weight you wish to achieve to improve your longevity. There is currently no hard and fast rule on what this should be. Most studies carried out on laboratory animals so far, with a calorie restriction of around 30 per cent, have found that longevity increased dramatically, sometimes by a staggering 100 per cent. Most anti-ageing researchers believe that a 5 to 10 per cent reduction from the ideal body weight to be a target for anyone seeking to promote longevity.

How to Calculate Your Ideal Body Weight and Live-Long Code Target Weight

For a female your ideal body weight is equal to 100 pounds plus 5 pounds for each inch you are above 5 feet. For example, if you are 5 feet 6 inches tall your ideal body weight is 130 pounds. Add a couple of pounds if you have a large frame and subtract a couple of pounds if you have a small frame. To calculate your Live-Long Code target weight, subtract 5 to 10 per cent from this ideal weight. The target Live-Long Code weight for the person in the example above is 118 to 122 pounds.

For a male, your ideal body weight is equal to 106 pounds plus 6 pounds for each inch you are above 5 feet. For example, if you are 6 feet tall, your ideal body weight is 178 pounds. Add five pounds if you have a large frame and subtract five pounds if you have a small frame. To calculate your target Live-Long Code weight, subtract 5 to 10 per cent from the ideal weight. The target Live-Long Code weight for the person in the example above is 161 to 171 pounds.

Height (feet and inches)	Male	Female
5' 0''	89–99 lb	88–92 lb
5' 1''	95–105 lb	93–97 lb
5' 2''	101–111 lb	98–102 lb
5' 3''	107–117 lb	103–107 lb
5' 4''	113–123 lb	108–112 lb
5' 5''	119–129 lb	113–117 lb
5' 6''	125–135 lb	118–122 lb
5' 7''	131-141 lb	123–127 lb
5' 8''	137–147 lb	128–132 lb
5' 9''	143–153 lb	133–137 lb
5' 10''	149–159 lb	138–142 lb
5' 11''	155–165 lb	143–147 lb
6' 0''	161–171 lb	148–152 lb
6' 1''	167–177 lb	153–157 lb
6' 2''	173–183 lb	158–162 lb
6' 3''	179–189 lb	163–167 lb
6' 4''	185–295 lb	168–172 lb
6' 5''	191–201 lb	173–177 lb
6' 6''	197–207 lb	178–182 lb

How to Reach Your Ideal Live-Long Code Weight

Most people in the western world are about 20 per cent above this Live-Long Code target weight. If you are already at this target weight level and feeling healthy, continue eating the same amount of food, but still take on board the nutrition advice in this chapter. Remember as well that quality is more important than quantity.

Always seek medical advice before embarking on any diet or weight reduction programme, especially if you have any medical conditions.

As you age, your metabolism slows down; consequently, people who continue to eat the same amount of food as earlier in life will slowly gain weight with age. We need less fuel as we age, so any extra will be stored as fat.

If you are looking to lose weight, you will need to burn approximately 3,500 calories to lose every pound of weight you are currently carrying. Losing one or two pounds a week is a good rate at which to lose weight. As you will be implementing the whole of the Live-Long Code Programme, and so may also be taking more exercise than you have been used to, you may well notice that you lose weight at a faster rate than this, which is fine; however, do not put pressure on yourself to lose weight fast.

There are only two ways that are safe and appropriate for losing weight and keeping it off. They are exercise and calorie restriction, both of which are part of the Live-Long Code. If you are currently consuming around 2,300 calories a day, by following the Live-Long Code Nutrition Programme you are likely to lose about 500 calories a day (3,500 calories a week). Add to this the Live-Long Code Exercise Programme, in which you will burn an additional 1,500 calories a week (based on three workouts at 500 calories a session). In total, you will lose about 5,000 calories a week, which is approximately equivalent to one and a half pounds a week.

In other words, all you have to do to lose 1 ½ pounds a week is consume 20 per cent fewer calories every day and exercise for about 30 minutes three times a week. In just 2 months, by sticking with the Live-Long Code Nutrition and Exercise Programme you would be likely to lose one stone. If you are very overweight, remember that it has probably taken you many years to gradually put that weight on. Be patient, and avoid starvation approaches and quick-fix diets; they generally don't work and are likely to have a rebound effect.

When you reach your target Live-Long Code weight, you will need around 2,000 calories a day, depending on your height, to maintain your weight. By eating the healthy foods recommended by the Live-Long Code Nutrition Plan and avoiding junk food, you will find that you can eat a lot of food without exceeding this target.

The keys for implementing a calorie restriction diet are:

- It should be executed slowly over time.
- It should include highly nutritious food and supplements to guard against malnutrition.
- It should be supervised by a doctor.

Optimum Nutrition

For many of us, the food that we eat represents more than just a source of nutrition. Food can also be a source of comfort, a recreational hobby, a means of family connection and a conduit to socialising. Because of this, nutrition and nutritional changes carry emotional challenges. Moreover, despite the burgeoning media interest in healthy eating, we are now seeing an increased rate of obesity in the Western world. Most worrying is the dramatic increase in childhood obesity – a trend which, if it continues, will lead to myriad problems for these people as they reach adulthood.

It wasn't until I was diagnosed with multiple sclerosis (MS) that I looked properly at my nutrition. I had been deluding myself that I had a good diet because I did eat a lot of nutritious food. However, I also ate a lot of poor-quality junk food but thought that the good foods were somehow compensating for this. Most people who come to my clinic believe that they have a reasonably healthy and balanced diet, but on closer inspection this rarely is the case. People are often confused about what a healthy eating plan is, and producers of substandard foods play their own part in trying to mislead the consumer.

Pure and simple, the food you put into your body every day has a huge influence on your health. When I changed my eating habits it took just eight short weeks for me to feel completely different in both mind and body. This is not, however, a temporary measure and my vitality has continued to grow as I have maintained this exceptionally good eating plan.

I researched what nutritional elements were for preventing illnesses such as heart disease, cancer, diabetes and neurological disorders, as well as a whole host of other conditions. The Live-Long Code Nutrition Plan draws together common aspects of all these food strategies and prepares your body for optimum health and longevity.

This plan is a key element of the Live-Long Code. It is now an accepted fact that nutrition plays a direct role in the development of a lot of illnesses and is therefore a contributory factor to, if not a direct cause of, many deaths. It is therefore common sense that the food that we eat provides a key to prolonging a healthy lifespan. Apart from the air we breathe, the only other source of healthy input into our bodies comes from what we eat and drink. I believe that although it can be challenging to correct your eating habits, when it comes to nutrition there should be no half measures and you really should endeavour to follow the nutrition plan to the full. This will ensure that a vital component of longevity – the fuel we are putting into our system – is optimised.

The Live-Long Code Nutrition Plan aims to help your body to regenerate itself and sustains your health by bombarding your body with nutrients. Many of the optimum food strategies for treating major health conditions are covered by this plan. There is broad medical consensus as to what foods are best for optimising health. This growing convergence of opinion from the world's leading nutritional scientists has led directly to the Live-Long Code Nutrition Plan, developed as it was from information derived from much evidence-based research carried out by the world's leading nutritional scientists.

The Free Radical Theory of Ageing and the Role of Antioxidant Foods

Earlier in the book we saw that Denham Harman MD from the University of Nebraska developed the free radical theory of ageing. According to this theory our bodies age because free radicals, or abnormal molecules that are missing an electron, cause instability by bonding with nearby 'normal' molecules. There are many things that accelerate the production of these free radicals, including chemical toxins, poor diet and smoking. Although we seek in this plan to minimise free radical damage, it is impossible to completely avoid it – basic acts of living such as breathing, eating and drinking all play a part in their production.

Harman recognised that free radicals are the main culprits that destroy cell structure. The best things we can do to prevent free radical damage are to cut down on the activities that produce excessive free radicals, such as smoking, exposure to toxins and eating junk food, and to bombard your body with a wide variety of antioxidants. The nutrients in antioxidants help your body to neutralise free radicals and hence fight against ageing and ill health. They are stable molecules that neutralise the free radicals by donating one of their own electrons to them. Antioxidants act like hunters, searching out free radicals and preventing them from causing the cellular and tissue damage that can ultimately lead to age-related diseases. We will look to a wide variety of antioxidants, obtainable from food and supplements, to help protect against free radical damage. The more important antioxidants include betacarotene, coenzyme Q10 and vitamins C and E. A fundamental aspect of the Live-Long Code Nutrition Plan is that it is very high in these important antioxidants.

The principles of the Live-Long Code Nutrition Plan are broadly accepted by leading medical authorities in both Western and Eastern medicine. The following are the main principles of the plan.

What to Eat

- Replace bad fats – saturated and trans fats – with good fats.
- Eliminate all processed foods containing trans fatty acids.
- Eliminate dairy products containing 1 per cent butterfat or more and replace with soya or rice milk.
- Eliminate refined carbohydrates, including sugar, white bread and pasta.
- Replace red and dark meat with healthier sources of protein.
- Consume large quantities of organic fruit and vegetables.

- Drink plenty of water and restrict alcohol consumption to a maximum of one glass of red wine a day.
- Replace coffee and tea with green tea.
- Replace refined table salt with healthy spices.

Although the Live-Long Code Nutrition Plan is based on much modern scientific evidence, it is remarkably similar to the diet of our ancient ancestors, which contained most of these elements.

Replace	With
Red and brown meat	Poultry, fish and vegetable protein
Butter	Organic extra virgin olive oil
Milk	Skimmed milk or organic soya milk
Chocolate	Raisins and dried fruit
Sugar	Moderate amounts of organic honey
Soft drinks	Fresh juices and water
Beer	Red wine (max one glass a day)
Coffee and tea	Green or jasmine tea
White bread	Wholemeal bread
Table salt	Spices

Altering the Eating Habits of a Lifetime

I have seen thousands of people at my clinic, and changing eating habits is one of the challenges to which many people have the most internal resistance. As mentioned earlier, food carries with it a great deal of emotional content; plus, most people's eating habits have been formed over an extended period of time, often going right back to childhood. In addition, because our knowledge of food has developed quickly in recent years, many of us were brought up with the misunderstanding that some foods now thought to be suboptimal are actually beneficial to us.

However, I do believe that altering eating habits is one of the most powerful things that you can do to optimise your health and extend your healthy lifespan. When you change your eating habits and feel the resulting surge of vitality and well being, you will find continuing to stick to the plan easier. If you think that the change required to your eating habits to follow the plan is dramatic, just think – the improvement in the way you feel will probably be equally dramatic!

When I changed my own diet I gave up many foods that I had previously adored. In order to achieve this I used many techniques to alter my behaviour around eating. These amazing techniques are explained in the next chapter, The Live-Long Code Detox, and they will support you.

The following table gives a comprehensive listing of many popular foods, along with guidance on how freely you should eat each food. Foods listed as a 'good choice' you are free to eat in any permissible amount. With foods that say 'avoid completely' you should do just that, as these foods are likely to actively slow your health recovery.

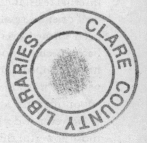

✓ = good choice
✗ = avoid completely
◆ = caution – limited intake
A = anti-cancer
B = high in antioxidants
C = antiviral
D = high in refined carbohydrates

◆	Alfalfa	A	Thought to protect against breast cancer and reduces inflammation, but avoid with auto-immune diseases
✓	Apple	A	Lowers cholesterol and relieves constipation
✓	Apricots	A	Used frequently by Chinese medicine to treat cancer, improves circulation, natural laxative
✓	Artichokes	B	Supports liver function and improves digestion
✓	Asparagus	B	Stimulates the kidneys
✓	Aubergine	B, C	Helps prevent strokes and haemorrhages. Protects against cholesterol damage
✓	Avocado	B	Good blood tonic
✗	Bagel	D	Eat only wholewheat bagels
✗	Baked beans	D	High in sugar
◆	Banana	C	Limit intake – high in potassium and has antibiotic qualities, but can be problematic for diabetics. Can cause acid residues
✓	Barley	A, B	Reduces cholesterol. Supports liver and digestive function
✓	Bean curd (tofu)	A, B, C	Helps to lower cholesterol
✗	Beef		High in saturated fat
✓	Beetroot	A, B	A rich source of vitamins and minerals. Supports detoxification and strengthens blood
✗	Biscuits	D	High in trans fats
✓	Black beans	A, B	Lowers cholesterol. Good source of fibre and protein
✓	Bok choi	A, B	Stimulates immunity and improves digestion
✓	Broccoli	A, B, C	Supports liver function and intestinal cleanser

✓	Brown rice		A healthier alternative to white rice, high in vitamins and minerals. Calms nervous system and lifts mood
✓	Brussels sprouts	A, B	Supports pancreatic function. Protects against a variety of cancers
✓	Buckwheat		High in fibre and protein
✓	Butter beans	A, B	Lowers cholesterol. Good source of fibre and protein
✓	Cabbage	A, B	Stimulates immunity and improves digestion
✗	Cakes	D	High in trans fats
✓	Carrots	A, B	High in beta carotene
✓	Cashew nuts	B	Only choose unsalted cashew nuts. Lowers cholesterol
✓	Cauliflower	A, B	Supports kidney and bladder function
✓	Celery	A, B	Supports digestion and lowers blood pressure
✗	Cereal bars	D	High in sugar and trans fats
✗	Cheese		High in saturated fat
✓	Cherries (fresh)	B	Strengthens immunity and relieves headaches
✓	Chicken		Choose only organic free-range chicken and eat only lean chicken breast
✗	Chicken nuggets		High in trans fats and saturated fats
✓	Chickpeas	B	Anti-inflammatory and supports digestive and kidney function. Excellent source of protein
◆	Chillies		Limit intake – can cause inflammation of the stomach
✓	Chives	A, B, C	Lowers cholesterol
✗	Chocolate	D	High in saturated fats
✗	Coffee		High in caffeine, which can cause a variety of health problems. Decaf coffee should also be avoided because of potentially harmful chemicals
✗	Cola drinks	D	Exceptionally high in sugar
✗	Commercial breakfast cereals	D	Generally avoid, as most contain excessive sodium, sugar and other refined carbohydrates
✓	Corn	A, B	High in good fats and supports nervous system function
✗	Cornflakes	D	High in sugar

✓	Courgette	B	Contains vitamins A, B and C and can alleviate bladder and kidney infections
✓	Cranberries	B, C	Supports bladder and kidney function
✗	Croissant	D	High in trans fats
✓	Cucumber	B	Supports digestion as well as kidney and bladder function
✗	Custard	D	High in sugar
✓	Dates	A	Used to treat respiratory conditions
✗	Diet soft drinks		Avoid completely – contains artificial sweeteners, which may damage the central nervous system
✗	Digestive biscuits	D	High in trans fats and sugar
✗	Duck		High in saturated fat
◆	Eggs		Limit to 4 eggs per week. Good source of protein, iron, selenium, vitamins B and D, but raises cholesterol. Only choose organic free-range eggs
✓	Fennel	A	Helps prevent blood clotting and supports digestive function
✓	Fish (oily)		High in omega-3 EFA and protects against a wide variety of conditions
✗	French fries		High in trans and saturated fats
◆	Fruit juice		Avoid commercial fruit juices; make your own juices from organic fruit
✓	Garlic	A, C	Lowers cholesterol, decongestant and prevents blood clotting
✓	Grapefruit	A, B	Lowers cholesterol, supports cardiovascular function. Fights allergies and throat and mouth infections
✓	Grapes	B	Good blood tonic
✓	Green beans	B	Boosts white blood cell count immunity
✗	Ham		High in saturated fat
✗	Hamburger		High in saturated fat and trans fats
◆	Honey		Moderate intake of organic honey is a good replacement for sugar
✓	Houmous	A	High in protein and fibre
✗	Ice cream	D	Contains dairy and high in sugar
✗	Jam	D	Exceptionally high in sugar

✗	Jelly	D	High in sugar
✓	Kale	A, B	Helps regulate hormones
✓	Kidney beans	A, B	Supports digestive function
✓	Kiwi	A, B	Used in Chinese medicine to treat cancer. Supports digestive function
✗	Lamb		High in saturated fat
✓	Leeks	B	Supports detoxification
✓	Lemon	A, B	Strengthens immune function
✓	Lentils	A	High in folic acid
✓	Lettuce		Rich in fibre and vitamins. Suports bones and joints
✓	Lime	A, B	Strengthens immune function
◆	Liquorice	A	Limit intake of real liquorice, has anti-cancer properties and kills bacteria. Avoid if experiencing raised blood pressure or pregnant. Supports digestive function. These benefits do not apply to liquorice sweets
✓	Mango	A, B, C	Antibacterial and immuno-boosting. Supports kidney and digestive function
✗	Marmalade	D	Exceptionally high in sugar
✗	Milk, full fat		High in saturated fat and weakens digestion
✗	Milk, semi-skimmed		High in saturated fat and weakens digestion
✓	Milk, skimmed		Permissible. Also consider organic soya milk
✗	Muffins	D	High in trans fats, saturated fats and sugar
✓	Mung beans	A, B	Good blood cleanser and supports detoxification
✓	Mushrooms	A	Shiitake mushrooms are used to treat a wide variety of conditions. Supports immunity
◆	Noodles		Choose only organic wholewheat noodles
✓	Oats	B	Good choice – high in antioxidants and lowers cholesterol. Some people are intolerant to oats, however, and if you experience bloating or digestive problems its best to avoid them
✓	Onions	A, B, C	Natural antibiotic. Supports detoxification
✓	Orange	A, B	High in vitamin C and supports digestion
✓	Orange juice		Good choice when juiced at home. Avoid processed juices

✓	Parsnips	A, B	Supports kidney and digestive function
✓	Pasta		Choose only organic wholewheat pasta
✓	Peach (fresh)	B	Supports detoxification, rich in minerals
✓	Peanuts (unsalted)		High in good fats, vitamins and minerals. Eat only unsalted peanuts
✓	Pear	B	High in iodine and benefits thyroid function. Supports digestion and detoxification
✓	Peas		Good source of vegetable protein. Source of calcium. Supports liver function
✓	Peppers	B	Good choice – high in antioxidants and vitamin C
✓	Pineapple	C	Suppresses inflammation. Antibacterial qualities
✓	Pinto beans	A, B	High in protein and dietary fibre
◆	Pitta bread		Eat only wholemeal pitta bread
✗	Pizza	D	Avoid completely – high in saturated fat
✓	Plum	C	Good source of fibre. Supports blood circulation and digestion
✗	Popcorn	D	High in salt and refined carbohydrates
✗	Pork		High in saturated fat
✓	Porridge	B	Lowers cholesterol. Some people are intolerant to oats, however, and if you experience bloating or digestive problems it is best to avoid them
◆	Potatoes	A	Limit intake – anti-cancer properties but as it raises insulin levels you should eat in moderation, particularly if trying to lose weight
✗	Pretzels	D	Avoid completely – high in salt and refined carbohydrates
✓	Prunes		High in fibre. Supports blood and central nervous system. Helps to lower cholesterol
✓	Pumpkin	A, B	High in beta carotene, protects against heart disease
✓	Radishes	B	Expectorant which reduces mucus and helps to clear sinuses. Supports digestion
✓	Raisins	B	High in vitamins and minerals

◆	Rhubarb	B	High in vitamins B, C, iron and calcium. Lowers cholesterol. Acidic, so avoid if dealing with kidney stones, gout, gallstones or cancer
✓	Rice	A, B	Choose only brown rice – high in vitamins, minerals and fibre. Lowers cholesterol and inhibits the development of kidney stones
✓	Rocket	A, B	Stimulates appetite and supports digestion
✓	Rye bread		High in dietary fibre and complex carbohydrates. Benefits the liver and supports digestion
✗	Salami	B	Avoid completely – high in saturated fat
◆	Salmon	B	Only eat wild salmon, as farmed salmon has been shown to contain cancer-causing polychlorinated biphenyls, or PCBs, that exceed health guidelines. Rich in omega-3 essential fatty acids. Boosts immunity
✓	Sardines	B	Good choice – high in omega-3 EFAs and protects against a wide variety of conditions
✗	Sausages		Avoid completely – high in saturated fat
✗	Scallops		Avoid completely – prone to toxic contamination
✓	Sesame seeds	B	Lowers cholesterol. Rich in omega-3 and -6 EFAs. Benefits cardiovascular and nervous systems
✓	Shallots	A, B	Protects against blood clotting
✗	Shellfish (prawn, crab, lobster)		Avoid completely – prone to toxic contamination
✗	Soft drinks		Avoid completely – contains extremely high amounts of refined sugar
✓	Soy beans	A, B, C	Helps to lower cholesterol
✓	Soya milk	A, B, C	Good choice – anti-cancer properties – only use organic soya milk
✓	Spaghetti		Choose only organic wholewheat spaghetti
✓	Spinach	A, B	High in beta carotene. Regulates blood pressure and supports immunity and bone health
✓	Spring onions	A, B, C	Helps prevent tumour and cancer formations. Supports digestion and blood circulation. Strengthens bones and joints
✗	Steak		High in saturated fat

✓	Strawberries	A, B, C	Good choice – antiviral and anti-cancer properties
✗	Stuffing, bread	D	High in saturated fats and trans fats
✗	Sugar	D	Avoid completely – causes a variety of health problems
✓	Sultanas	B	High in vitamins and minerals
✓	Sweet potato	B	High in beta carotene
◆	Tea, English		Limit intake – high caffeine content
✓	Tea, green	A, B	Excellent choice – high in antioxidants and has anti-cancer properties
✓	Tea, jasmine	A, B	Excellent choice – high in antioxidants and has anti-cancer properties
✓	Tofu	A, B, C	Helps to lower cholesterol
✓	Tomato	A, B	Antiseptic. Reduces liver inflammation
✓	Trout	B	Good choice – high in omega-3 EFA and protects against a wide variety of conditions
✓	Tuna	B	Good choice – high in omega-3 EFA and protects against a wide variety of conditions
✓	Turkey		Good choice – low in saturated fat. Only eat the white meat of turkey
✗	Veal		Avoid completely – high in saturated fat
◆	Vinegar		Limit intake, particularly if suffering from digestive disorders. Use lemon juice as an alternative
✗	Waffles	D	Avoid completely – high in trans fats
✓	Watercress	A, B	Good choice – antioxidant and anti-cancer properties. Stimulates the appetite and acts as a tonic
✓	Watermelon	A, B	Good source of potassium
◆	Wheat	A	High incidence of intolerance towards wheat, so avoid if you experience bloating or digestive problems. If not, wheat does have good anti-cancer properties
✗	White bread	D	High in trans fats and refined carbohydrates
✓	Wholemeal bread		Good choice – but avoid if you show signs of intolerance – bloating, indigestion, etc.
◆	Yoghurt	A	Limit – only choose live organic low saturated fat varieties. Antibacterial and anti-cancer properties. Contains acidophilus bacteria

The Principles of the Live-Long Code Nutrition Plan

Good Fats Versus Bad Fats

Many people think that all fat is simply bad for us, but in fact there are many different kinds of fat, some of which are good for you – indeed essential – although others are considered bad. But which is which? It is very important that you understand the answer to this question as, to put it simply, 'bad' fats will age you and potentially cause serious damage to your health, and 'good' fats will preserve and protect your health.

There are two types of fat that are generally accepted as being bad for us: trans fats and saturated fats. Because there is established evidence against both of these fats, the Live-Long Code Nutrition Plan encourages the reduction of saturated fat intake and the complete elimination of trans fats.

Possibly because trans fats have such a bad reputation, processed-food manufacturers sometimes use different terms to confuse the consumer. Trans fats are sometimes called hydrogenated vegetable oil or trans fatty acids. Under these names, trans fats can be found in many processed foods, including biscuits, cakes, margarines, many domestic cooking oils and, disturbingly, baby food. Thankfully these fats are now widely accepted as being so bad that they are starting to disappear from the shelves of some supermarkets, and in the US whole cities and states are starting to ban their use. If you look at the label of any processed food that you buy (and hopefully that will soon be less) and see hydrogenated or trans fats on the label, put it right back on the shelf.

Trans fats are made through a process called hydrogenation. This process combines heat and pressure to add several hydrogen atoms to liquid oil over several hours until it converts to a semisolid state. Although this hydrogenation process helps to prevent the oil from becoming rancid, it also destroys most of its nutritional value. Let's make no bones about it: the purpose of this process is to allow manufacturers to make their products more cheaply.

The hydrogenation process also produces residues of a variety of toxic metals that accumulate in our bodies' cells and central nervous system, where they can act to poison enzyme systems and alter cellular functions. Extended exposure to this can endanger your health and cause a whole host of problems.

Because trans or hydrogenated fats are not natural, our bodies are not capable of digesting them properly. This effectively makes them poisonous. The trans fat content of human red blood cells has been shown to be as high as 20 per cent. It is safe to assume that most other cellular membranes in the human body also contain high percentages of them. If they are indeed poisonous, this is not a reassuring thought.

When you consume trans fats, your cellular membranes become weaker or damaged, which alters the way in which healthy nutrients travel across the membrane. This can result in a variety of diseases as toxic chemicals can more easily invade the cells. Ultimately the result is poor organ function, damaged immunity and a dramatic increase in your risk of disease – in short, ageing.

Trans fats also inhibit the body's ability to eliminate cholesterol. Under normal circumstances, the liver turns any excess cholesterol into bile and transfers it to the gall bladder before it is moved to the small intestine. Trans fats block this normal conversion of cholesterol, which ultimately results in elevated cholesterol levels in the blood. This causes an increase in the amount of low-density lipoproteins (LDLs, or bad cholesterol), one of the chief contributors to arterial and heart disease. Trans fats also suppress lower high-density lipoproteins (HDLs, or good cholesterol), which under normal circumstances would act to protect the heart and cardiovascular system from the negative effects of the LDLs.

Trans fats also increase inflammation and suppress the production of anti-inflammatory hormones. As a result we become more vulnerable to inflammatory conditions such as arthritis, colitis, asthma and bronchitis, as well as allergic reactions, high blood pressure and suppressed immune function.

There is significant scientific evidence that trans fats contribute to heart disease, cancer, diabetes, reproductive problems and obesity. A Harvard Medical School study followed more than 85,000 women over eight years and found that major dietary sources of trans fats, such as margarine, were significantly associated with higher risks of coronary heart disease.

So be sure to read the labels on packaged foods and always avoid those with hydrogenated or partially hydrogenated oil. Because most food labels do not include the amount of trans fats on the nutritional information panel, it is wise to look for partially hydrogenated vegetable oil. If this is listed as one of the first three ingredients, it usually indicates that the product contains substantial amounts of trans fats.

Saturated fats are found in common foods such as milk, butter, cream, cheese, chocolate, coconut and red meat. When we cut down our intake of saturated fat, cholesterol levels drop accordingly. It is widely thought that is it wise to minimise intake of saturated fats, as they play a role in raising bad cholesterol (LDL) and increasing the risk of cardiovascular disease.

Saturated fats are nonessential to our bodies and our diet. Animal fats found in dairy and meat are high in a particular saturated fat called stearic acid. Although stearic acid may not raise LDL (bad cholesterol) levels, it does increase inflammation, which is acknowledged as a factor in cardiovascular disease development as well as cancer and many other diseases.

Saturated fats are solid at room temperature and can replace the more positive unsaturated fats in the body's cells, which remain liquid at room temperature and become incorporated into cell membranes. This can make the cell membranes more rigid, causing malfunctions, including insulin resistance.

Studies have revealed that when we replace saturated fat with unsaturated oils, we can achieve up to a 65 per cent reduction in heart disease deaths. Treatment with statin drugs, which lower LDL cholesterol, seem only to be half as effective as this dietary change because the drugs don't address all the risks.

There is strong evidence to suggest that many 'good' fats actually reduce the risk of stroke and heart attack. Good fats help with sugar and insulin metabolism and as a consequence assist in weight management.

Good fats include monounsaturated fats, found in extra virgin olive and canola oils, nuts and avocados. Monounsaturated fats actually lower total and bad LDL cholesterol, while maintaining levels of good HDL cholesterol, which carries cholesterol from artery walls and delivers it to the liver for removal.

Two types of good fatty acids — omega-3 and omega-6 — which are essential for our cells to function normally, cannot be made by our bodies and must be obtained from foods or supplements in our diets. They are called essential fatty acids (EFAs), and they are building blocks for many of our bodies' hormones. There is evidence that they have been helpful to many people with conditions including allergies, anaemia, arthritis, cancer, candida, chronic fatigue, depression, diabetes, eczema, heart disease, multiple sclerosis, premenstrual syndrome (PMS), psoriasis, sluggish metabolism and viral infections.

Omega-3 fatty acids are polyunsaturated fats found in coldwater fish, canola oil, flaxseed, walnuts and almonds. Studies have proven that people who eat more omega-3s have a lower risk of heart disease and diabetes. One study established that healthy women who ate fish at least five times a week had a 45 per cent lower risk of developing heart disease. Another study showed that men who had experienced a heart attack, when randomly assigned fish oil supplements had a 53 per cent reduction in mortality in comparison to those given a placebo.

There is also evidence to suggest that omega-3 oils help to prevent and treat depression, arthritis and asthma, as well as a number of other conditions.

Omega-6 oils are typically found in vegetables and grains and a deficiency of this essential fatty acid can result in autoimmune problems, eczema, hypertension, inflammation and skin problems.

To make sure you obtain the appropriate amounts of essential fatty acids, the Live-Long Code Nutrition Plan recommends at least three servings of oily fish a week, together with adequate portions of leafy green vegetables. If you dislike fish, another option is to take flaxseed, canola and soy oils as well as walnuts and soy beans. If you do not eat fish, I would also suggest that you take a good-quality 1,000 mg fish oil supplement a day.

Remember to store your oils properly after opening. If they are not in lightproof bottles you should keep them out of direct light, as this makes the oil putrefy.

Going Dairy-Free

The dairy industry has put a lot of effort into trying to convince us that we cannot survive as a species unless we drink the milk of another animal. If anyone claimed that you needed pig milk, horse milk or ape milk to survive you would immediately recognise how silly that sounds. So why do we think that we need cows' milk? Going dairy-free will change how you look and how you feel as well as adding years to your life. It is scientifically established that full-fat dairy products are detrimental to our health.

Cows produce milk for their calves, which are supposed to feed on their mothers' milk until they are weaned from it. If an adult cow drank the pasteurised milk from another cow it would be likely to die within weeks. Humans are the only mammals that by choice drink milk once we have reached adulthood, not to mention drinking the milk of a completely different species that is much bigger than us. Many people consume vast quantities of dairy each day and are convinced that they are doing themselves good, but the reality is that our digestive system is not designed to break down a food that is meant to nurse the young of another species. Remember also that cows are frequently exposed to large amounts of steroids and antibiotics, which can get into their milk. Most cows also graze on pesticide-infested grass, and milk can also carry pus from cows that have mastitis, which is treated with antibiotics.

The fat in whole milk, which becomes highly condensed in foods such as cream, ice cream, cheese and butter, is the most saturated of animal fats. This fat, which dominates the typical Western diet, is probably the biggest single contributor to saturated-fat overload and can therefore be considered responsible for the exceptionally high rates of cardiovascular disease in Western societies.

Cows' milk has four times the protein and only half the carbohydrate content of human milk; pasteurisation destroys the natural enzyme required to digest its heavy protein content. This excess milk protein therefore putrefies in the human digestive tract, clogging the intestines with sticky sludge, some of which seeps into the bloodstream. As the sludge accumulates with daily consumption of dairy products, the body forces some of it out through the skin (manifesting in acne and blemishes) and the lungs (contributing to catarrh), while the rest of it forms mucus and breeds infections, causes allergic reactions and stiffens joints with calcium deposits. Many cases of chronic asthma, allergies, ear infections and acne have been totally cured simply by the elimination of all dairy products from the diet.

When I gave up dairy in 1998 I noticed a huge change in the way I felt within just a few weeks. I had lived with bad sinus problems for as long as I could remember, but within weeks of giving up dairy my sinus problems had gone and have never come back.

One concern that a lot of people may have when thinking about eliminating dairy is that they might not consume enough calcium and so may be vulnerable to osteoporosis. The reality is that osteoporosis rates are much lower in societies where people do not eat dairy products. The high protein content of dairy products tends to leach calcium from our bodies; for every gram of protein that you eat, you will lose up to 2 mg of calcium in your urine. In addition, cows' milk also contains a large amount of phosphorus, which combines with calcium in the digestive tract and tends to block calcium assimilation. This means that although cows' milk has high levels of calcium, it is not necessarily as good a source as other more digestible foods such as broccoli, kale, sesame seeds, dates, figs, prunes, kelp and sardines. Remember that cows get their calcium simply from eating grass.

Refined Carbohydrates – Man-Made Poison

Refined carbohydrates are in fact anything but refined! These insulin-producing, fat-causing, energy-destroying, stomach-bloating foods have been artificially created by man.

Refined carbohydrates include foods such as:

- Baked goods: muffins, doughnuts, pastries, cookies, cakes.
- White flour and white-flour products such as white bread and bagels.
- Snack foods: candy, crisps, pretzels.
- Sweetened dairy products: ice cream, chocolate milk.
- Drinks: pop/soda, juice.
- Processed grain products: pasta made from white flour, white rice, rice cakes, many breakfast cereals.

Refined carbohydrates have little or no nutritional value and are usually detrimental to our health. They are found in most processed foods and they wreak havoc with your digestion and turn your blood sugar levels into a rollercoaster of highs and lows. This in turn can cause a host of things to happen throughout your body. One particularly nasty culprit is high-fructose corn syrup, which is found in a wide variety of foods including ketchup, juices and breakfast cereals. The Live-Long Code Nutrition Plan recommends that you avoid all processed foods for this reason, amongst others. White flour is also a refined carbohydrate; it is recommended that you avoid white bread, cakes and biscuits made from white flour.

When you remove refined carbohydrates from your diet you may experience cravings as your body gets used to coming off the blood-sugar rollercoaster. However, the more you reduce your refined carbohydrate intake, the less you will crave it. When you remove it from your body you will find that you have fewer blood sugar swings and more consistent energy. Your taste buds will also return to normal and you will start tasting your food properly again. Food will start to taste like it used to in 'the good old days' – the reality being that natural food always tasted good and it was just your taste buds that had been suppressed by artificially intense-tasting food.

Refined Carbohydrate	Replace With
White bread	Wholegrain or rye bread
Regular pasta	Wholewheat pasta
Ramen noodles	Buckwheat noodles
White rice	Brown rice
Concentrated fruit juice	Fruit
Breakfast cereals	Oatmeal

Sugar – The Silent Killer

We consume up to 15 times more sugar today than we did 100 years ago; around 150 g a day. Most of us have no idea that we are consuming so much sugar as it is concealed in a wide variety of processed foods under a number of different names – corn syrup, dextrose, fructose, lactose and sucrose, to name but a few.

This huge increase in refined sugar consumption has mirrored the dramatic rise in the incidence of heart disease. At the beginning of the twentieth century heart disease was relatively rare in the Western world, but now it accounts for almost half of all deaths. Scientific studies are starting to indicate that sugar is a contributory factor in this dramatic rise, as well as in many other degenerative and ageing diseases. So if you are concerned with living longer, the case for avoiding sugar is quite compelling.

Avoiding or reducing sugar can help you avoid elevated blood-insulin levels. High insulin levels promote the formation of fat in the body and consequently increases your risk of heart attack. In a Finnish study, the participants with the highest insulin levels were three times as likely to have a heart attack as the ones with the lowest insulin levels. High sugar consumption can also cause diabetes, which in turn increases the risk of heart disease.

Ten Reasons to Avoid Sugar
- It can suppress immune function and impair your defences against infectious disease.

- It upsets the mineral balance in your body, causing chromium and copper deficiency and interfering with the absorption of calcium and magnesium.
- It can produce a significant rise in total cholesterol, triglycerides and bad cholesterol and a decrease in good cholesterol, leading to a dramatically increased risk of heart disease.
- It can feed cancer cells; studies have connected high suga consumption with the development of cancers of the breast, ovaries, prostate, rectum, pancreas, biliary tract, lung, gall-bladder and stomach.
- It can cause many gastrointestinal tract problems, including indigestion, malabsorption in patients with functional bowel disease, increased risk of Crohn's disease and ulcerative colitis.
- It can impair the structure of your DNA.
- Sugar intake has been found to be higher in people with Parkinson's disease.
- It can increase kidney size and contribute to the formation of kidney stones.
- Diets high in sugar increase free radicals, contributing to disease and oxidative stress.
- It can induce abnormal metabolic processes and promote chronic degenerative diseases.

Artificial Sweeteners

'There are known knowns. These are things we know that we know. There are known unknowns. That is to say, there are things that we know we don't know. But there are also unknown unknowns. There are things we don't know we don't know.' Donald Rumsfeld, US Secretary of Defense and former CEO of Searle, developers of aspartame

A lot of people, in an effort to be healthy, choose diet foods and drinks, many of which contain artificial sweeteners that give a sweet taste without the calorie content of sugar. Artificial sweeteners such as aspartame (also known and sometimes listed on labels as E951) and saccharine are now well established and generally accepted. However, man-made artificial sweeteners have been linked with numerous health problems, and so I would strongly recommend that you avoid them.

It took the US Food and Drug Administration 16 years to approve aspartame because of serious concerns about its safety. According to top doctors and researchers, aspartame can cause headaches, memory loss, vision loss, seizures, coma and cancer. It worsens or mimics the symptoms of diseases and conditions such as fibro-myalgia, MS, lupus, Attention Deficit Disorder, diabetes, Alzheimer's disease, chronic fatigue and depression. Further, aspartame releases free methyl alcohol. This can result in methanol or wood alcohol poisoning, which affects the brain and can cause addiction. It is somewhat disturbing to reflect that aspartame is used in the kind of processed foods that are promoted as healthy options. Don't be fooled! This stuff is potentially deadly. It is also worth noting that after 16 years it was Searle's then chief executive, Donald Rumsfeld, who finally received FDA approval for this substance. Rumsfeld later became George Bush's Secretary of Defense. I think that probably says more than enough.

A side effect of artificial sweeteners is that they create strong carbohydrate cravings and as a result they actually tend to cause weight gain; ironic when you consider that a lot of people choose them in an effort to *lose* weight.

There are many reasons to avoid artificial sweeteners. A good alternative to sugar is a moderate amount of organic honey and the natural sweetness of fruit.

Choose Healthy Sources of Protein

There are healthier ways to consume protein than eating red meat, which has been linked with a variety of cancers including cancers of the breast, colon, stomach, lymph system, bladder and prostate. As red meat has high levels of saturated fat, it is also associated with cardiovascular disease. It can therefore be considered to be a risk factor for just about all the top killer diseases of modern society.

Some people believe that our ancient ancestors ate large quantities of red meat, but the idea of the meat-eating caveman is a bit of a fallacy and images of our ancestors hunting woolly mammoth are largely a fiction created by the movies. The reality is that we developed as a species without eating large quantities of red meat; in our distant history our diet came for the most part from wild plants, occasionally supplemented by small game and fish.

Humans are more herbivore than carnivore. Our closest living relatives in the animal world, apes, are 98 per cent vegetarian and our own digestive systems have been designed to cater for a predominantly vegetarian diet. Studies have shown that if people eat the foods that dominated the meals of our Stone Age ancestors, the incidence of a variety of cancers and other killer conditions decreases significantly.

Red meat is unhealthy partly because its saturated fat content contributes to heart disease and atherosclerosis. Also, the cooking process causes carcinogens to form; some researchers believe that this alone could be a direct cause of colon cancer.

Another factor that should be borne in mind when considering red meat is that when a cow is being slaughtered, adrenalin goes through its body and is passed on to us through the meat when it arrives on our plate. So when we eat the animal's flesh we are literally consuming its fear and terror.

Animals raised for meat are also exposed to hormones, chemicals and toxins, and sometimes questionable food during their lives. We are then exposed to some of these elements when we eat their flesh. All of these factors, together with the recent spate of health scares associated with eating the meat of various animals, make a compelling argument for the avoidance of red meat.

Healthier Alternatives to Red Meat

The meats favoured by the Live-Long Code Nutrition Plan include oily fish such as salmon, tuna and mackerel and the white meat of organic free-range chicken and turkey. In addition, the programme recommends non-animal foods that are superior sources of protein.

We know that oily fish provides omega-3 fatty acids, which are critical for maintaining a healthy heart and immune system. The omega-3 fat in fish is a platelet inhibitor that prevents platelets forming clots in the coronary arteries and elsewhere, and helps lower bad cholesterol levels.

Oily fish is probably the best alternative to red meat, but the white meat from organic free-range chicken and turkey is also a good choice as it is lower in calories and fat, and actually higher in protein, than red meat. Try to choose organically reared chicken and turkey to minimise your exposure to conventional pesticides and fertilizers. Also, remember that the white meat is by far the healthiest, and always remove the skin before cooking.

If you are a vegetarian, you will not want to eat meat at all. This is fine, but you still have to make sure you are getting the right foods. It sometimes surprises me to hear how much junk food vegetarian clients of mine eat. And it amazes me that vegetarians frequently don't eat enough vegetables, but instead replace meat by overconsuming dairy products. As we have seen, the Live-Long Code Nutrition Plan recommends avoiding dairy products. You also need to ensure that you are getting adequate omega-3, from flaxseed or an alternative supplement.

Replacing animal protein with vegetable protein can have the additional benefit of giving you more antioxidants, vitamins and minerals. Also, vegetarian meat substitutes are often soya based and there is growing evidence that soya beans offer significant benefits for longevity. For example, studies show that if you eat just five grams of soya protein a day you can lower your blood cholesterol by 10 per cent. Studies also indicate that soya foods like tofu can help to strengthen bones and reduce the risk of heart disease and breast, prostate and colon cancer, and scientists now believe that flavones found in soybeans may actually inhibit the growth of cancer cells.

Nuts are a good source of protein for non-meat eaters and also provide excellent antioxidant benefits. Almonds and soya nuts are especially good as they are high in heart-protecting monounsaturated fats. Just be careful to avoid salted nuts.

Eat Organic Fruit and Vegetables

Fruit and vegetables are an extremely healthy food choice. They are crammed full of nutrients and a diet high in fruit and vegetables will add years to your life by significantly protecting you against heart disease, cancer, stroke and hypertension. Vegetables are one of the main sources of dietary antioxidants, which, as we have seen, protects against cellular damage and disease.

Of course our bodies have their own built-in immune system, but it is our food that supplies the protective 'ammunition' for the system. It therefore makes a lot of sense to load up on antioxidant-rich food rather than empty calories, and the most antioxidant-rich foods are fruit and vegetables. A recent survey of 30,000 people conducted in the UK found that consumption of fruit and vegetables was positively correlated with all the indicators of good health.

With the Live-Long Code Nutrition Plan you will aim to eat at least five portions of organic fruit and vegetables a day. These foods will turbo-charge your health with powerful supernutrients.

What About Juicing?

Juicing does have its benefits; if you don't like eating certain fruit and vegetables it provides a means by which you can get some benefits in a form that you find more palatable. Consuming fruit and vegetables in juice form also allows these powerful foods to be easily and rapidly digested. However, it is worth bearing in mind that digestion starts in the mouth, where some of the most important digestive enzymes are found. The Chinese have a phrase, 'you should drink your food and eat your drink', which means that you should spend time chewing your food slowly and properly before you swallow it. The advantage of this approach over juicing is that some of the beneficial plant enzymes that tend to be lost in the juicing process, particularly with lower-cost home juicers, remain in your body. Chewing your food until it is almost liquefied therefore gives you all the benefits of juicing. So if you eat properly then there is really no need to juice your food.

Drinking from the Fountain of Youth

The human body is made up of around 60 per cent water and is in need of constant replenishment. Our lungs expel an average of three cups of water each day just through breathing. Also, you can lose up to a litre of water through normal sweating throughout the day, and if you exercise this increases significantly. Of course a lot of water is also lost through urination; if you make half a dozen trips to the bathroom during the day, six cups of water have been lost.

Water is a major source of energy and is vitally important to survival; while we can survive many weeks without food, we can last only a few days without water. Dehydration (lack of water) is a condition that occurs when there is not enough water for the body to carry out its normal functions. Even mild dehydration – as little as 1 to 2 per cent of your body weight – can sap your energy and make you feel tired. Some of the symptoms of dehydration include:

- Excessive thirst.
- Fatigue.
- Headache.
- Dry mouth.
- Little or no urination.
- Muscle weakness.
- Dizziness.
- Lightheadedness.

The US Institute of Medicine recommends that men should consume three litres of water a day and women should consume two litres a day. Do, however, try to stop drinking three hours before you retire for the evening, unless you really feel that you are getting dehydrated. Sleep is also vitally important to your health and drinking water late in the evening can cause sleep disturbance.

Where we get our water from is the next thing to consider. Despite all the assurances we are given, unfiltered tap water is not a good source as it usually contains residues of harmful chemicals such as benzene, pesticides and disinfectant by-products. Chemicals seep into our water supplies from waste-disposal sites, and pesticides are swept into lakes and streams from nearby land. Most mineral waters are not recommended either, as they often contain such high levels of radioactivity, nitrates and other pollutants that they would be illegal if they came out of a tap. A good approach is to filter your water through a standard charcoal filter, which will remove most of the harmful substances. You could also invest in a point-of-use filter, which is installed at the kitchen sink so that all the water you use is filtered.

It is a good idea to boil your water and drink it warm, rather than drinking direct from the fridge, as this is thought to be more beneficial to digestion; in Chinese medicine cold water is thought to put a strain on your digestive system, as your body has to work hard to heat it up. Bear in mind that warm water combats dehydration just as well as cold water.

What about soft drinks and alcohol? Most soft drinks contain refined carbohydrates, which, as discussed, have a hugely detrimental effect on our bodies. Alcohol rapidly dehydrates the body. When you are hung over you are actually suffering from the effects of dehydration. In general alcohol is not considered beneficial to healthy longevity. There is, however, one exception, which has become known as the French Paradox.

The French Paradox

If a glass of Pinot Noir or Cabernet Sauvignon is your pleasure then you might be doing yourself more good than harm. A number of scientific studies have found that certain compounds in red wine may actually benefit your health. But just how beneficial is it, and how much (or how little) should one drink to get the full health effect?

Despite its alcohol content it is thought that red wine has helpful properties, most particularly in the form of resveratrol. This is a chemical compound found in the skin of grapes and other plants that acts as a powerful antioxidant, protecting the cells in your body from free radical damage. Resveratrol has been touted as a break-through discovery in the world of anti-ageing medicine. Studies have established that when laboratory animals are given high doses of resveratrol, the result is similar to the results of the calorie restriction diet.

However, resveratrol is not on the Live-Long Code supplements list. In time I'm sure it will be, but although scientific studies suggest that a high intake of resveratrol is necessary, currently it is sold in quite small doses and taking the large amounts of resveratrol recommended by the studies is financially unviable. Until resveratrol can realistically become one of the Live-Long Code supplements, I recommend that you take one glass of red wine a day. This is in line with recent studies, which have shown a close relationship between moderate drinking of red wine and a healthy heart. White wine and other forms of alcohol do not have the same benefits and indeed are generally considered harmful. Research has suggested that daily consumption of a single glass of red wine gives 13 per cent more protection against cancer when compared with non-drinkers.

Replace Coffee with Alternatives – And Why You Should

Caffeine, most often consumed in coffee or tea, is technically an insecticide, from the same family of drugs as morphine and cocaine – neurotoxins. In other words, caffeine is harmful to the nervous system. It is also a powerful diuretic, which means that it robs your body of much-needed water and places a strain on your kidneys and liver.

Some Facts about Caffeine
- Caffeine affects the central nervous system, brain, lungs, heart, muscles and digestive system, raises blood pressure and increases heart rate.
- Caffeine increases stomach acid.
- Caffeine works on the urinary system to increase urine flow, which can irritate the bladder.

- Caffeine increases the release of adrenalin and can thus raise anxiety levels and cause panic.
- Caffeine increases the amount of calcium excreted in your urine.
- Caffeine causes insomnia.
- Caffeine can cause gastrointestinal upsets, including constipation and diarrhea.
- Caffeine increases stomach acid secretion. The stomach acids back up into the oesophagus and produce heartburn.
- Caffeine reduces iron absorption.

Consuming caffeine creates a vicious circle. As it is a stimulant it affects sleep patterns, which will then adversely affect your health recovery. When you are deprived of sleep and tired, it is tempting to drink more caffeine just to keep yourself awake. And so the disturbed sleep patterns continue, and the tiredness continues . . . This is the caffeine rollercoaster, which does little to support your health recovery.

Coffee lowers blood sugar and stems the flow of blood to the brain, which can cause palpitations and anxiety. Most decaffeinated coffee is unfortunately not such a good alternative, as it contains harmful chemicals such as turpentine and formaldehyde.

Green and jasmine tea are excellent choices as a substitute for tea or coffee. Drinking green tea after a meal is considered to be an excellent aid to digestion. Scientific research in both Asia and the West is currently providing hard evidence for the health benefits long anecdotally associated with drinking green tea. In 1994 the *Journal of the National Cancer Institute* published the results of an epidemiological study indicating that drinking green tea reduced the risk of oesophageal cancer in men and women by nearly 60 per cent. In another recent study, University of Purdue researchers concluded that a compound in green tea inhibits the growth of cancer cells. There is also research indicating that drinking green tea improves the ratio of good to bad cholesterol.

Jasmine tea, made from green tea leaves combined with fresh jasmine flowers, contains all the goodness of green tea and more.

Research studies have shown that laboratory animals live up 20 per cent longer when jasmine tea is added to their drinking water. The winning components of jasmine tea are its artery-cleansing flavonoids and high antioxidant levels; many studies have shown the potential role of tea flavonoids in cancer prevention, including cancers of the lung, breast, prostate, bladder, stomach and colon. Flavonoids have also been shown to be effective in helping to prevent heart disease and stroke.

Plain old English tea, unfortunately, does not seem to have the same health benefits. The principal difference is that jasmine and green teas have not been oxidised and have therefore retained the optimum quantity of flavonoids. It is recommended that you avoid regular tea – and coffee – and drink up to three cups of green or jasmine tea a day instead.

Replace Refined Table Salt with Healthy Spices

Salt is important for proper bodily function, but when consumed to excess it can lead to a whole host of health problems. We need approximately 500 mg of dietary sodium (salt) a day to meet our body's needs. By following the Live-Long Code Nutrition Plan, you will achieve this easily without needing to add any table salt or other forms of sodium.

By adding table salt to food, the average person consumes 15 times the required daily level, which can lead to high blood pressure, mineral deficiencies, heart attacks, strokes, kidney failure and a myriad of other conditions. Interestingly, overconsumption of sodium can cause a similar response to when we get a fright and the nervous system gets a rush of adrenalin. This response can lead to a heightened state of stress that can last for months or even years.

Most foods contain sodium as a part of their normal chemical composition. Ingredients such as baking powder, baking soda, soy sauce, pickles and olives contain significant amounts of sodium. Many processed foods also contain large amounts of salt in various forms – monosodium glutamate, sodium phosphate, sodium nitrite and sodium benzoate, to name just a few.

With the Live-Long Code Nutrition Plan, you will be avoiding processed foods and so will get adequate sodium supplies from natural sources. If you wish to season food to add taste you can choose from any of the following healthy alternatives:

Basil, bay leaves, cayenne, cinnamon, cloves, cumin, curry leaf, dill seed, fennel, garlic, ginger, horseradish, mustard seed, parsley, paprika, pepper, saffron, sesame seed, Szechuan pepper, thyme, tamarind, turmeric.

Supplements

Calorie restriction is an important component of the Live-Long Code Programme, so you need to address its potential pitfalls. When you are restricting calories you need to be very sure that you are getting enough of all the right nutrients that are vital for optimum healthy function. To get the right level of these nutrients through food alone, however, would require a high-calorie diet. It's a catch-22; a high-calorie diet leads to excess weight, but anything less provides nutrients in suboptimal anti-ageing quantities. That's where nutritional supplementation comes in. Taking supplements enables you to follow a calorie restriction programme and still consume the optimum level of nutrients.

A number of vitamins are required in small amounts for good nutrition. These are the fat-soluble vitamins A, D, E and K, the water-soluble B vitamins, and vitamin C. Most processed foods are depleted of vitamins, which often results in our bodies being starved of these vital nutrients. Deficiency results in a number of symptoms, including fatigue, weakness and loss of appetite. Vitamin A deficiency is associated with eye problems such as dry eyes and even blindness. Vitamin B is particularly important for carbohydrate metabolism. Severe vitamin B deficiency can cause symptoms such as mental confusion, paralysis and even heart failure. Vitamin C deficiency can lead to very poor healing recovery after injury, as well as lowered immunity.

The soils in which plants are grown for consumption have

become increasingly depleted of a number of vital nutrients, which means that food plants are often lacking these nutrients. Chemical fertilizers are very effective at stimulating crop growth even in nutrient-poor soils; the resultant food crops and vegetables appear to prosper but they are often lacking in the full range of minerals and vitamins.

The best way to consume vitamins is through a high-quality and varied organic diet, following the Live-Long Code Nutrition Plan. However, the following supplement programme is part of the Live-Long Code Nutrition Plan as there is gathering scientific evidence that these supplements lend support in protecting against many illnesses.

Supplement	Daily Dosage
Spirulina	6,000 mg
Vitamin B complex	50 mg
Vitamin C	2,000–10,000 mg
Vitamin D	5000 IU
Vitamin E	1,000 mg
Zinc	30 mg
Chromium	50 mg
Selenium	200 mcg
Coenzyme Q10	400 mg
L-carnosine	500 mg
MSM	2,000 mg

What These Supplements Can Do for Your Health

Spirulina

Spirulina is the most nutrition-dense food – animal or plant – known to man, and offers many nutrients that are lacking in most people's diets. It is the richest whole-food source of betacarotene (vitamin A), a natural antioxidant that offers powerful protection against free radical damage.

Spirulina is 25 times richer in this nutrient than raw carrots. Spirulina is also the richest whole-food source of vitamin B12, which provides energy and is essential for normal growth and neurological function.

The GLA (gammalinolenic acid) found in spirulina supports normal blood cholesterol and blood pressure, as well as normal joint function, premenstrual stress and skin health. The other minerals it contains are essential for healthy skin and bones.

Spirulina has twice the protein level of its nearest rival, the soybean, and at least three times that of beef, fish or eggs. The protein make-up of spirulina has a superior complete amino acid profile, containing all eight essential amino acids and 10 non-essential amino acids in the correct proportions. It is the most digestible form of protein available and the amino acids in it are delivered in an essentially 'free form' state for almost instantaneous assimilation.

Spirulina helps protect the immune system, reduces cholesterol and aids the absorption of minerals. It has been used in the treatment of diabetes, glaucoma, liver problems and cancer. For people with hypoglycaemia, a spirulina supplement can help regulate blood sugar levels.

Research at the Osaka Institute of Public Health in Japan has shown that spirulina promotes the activation of natural cancer-fighting substances in the body. In this clinical study volunteers over 40 years of age were given 50 ml of a spirulina extract and the levels of natural cancer-fighting substances in their blood were measured. The results showed that spirulina significantly increased the tumour-killing ability of the body's natural killer cells (NK cells). Also, surprisingly and interestingly, this beneficial activity continued for between 12 and 24 weeks after volunteers stopped taking the spirulina.

The recommended dosage of spirulina is 6,000 mg a day.

Vitamin B

The B vitamins, collectively known as B-complex, work together as a team. They perform a whole host of valuable functions: they promote healthy nerves, skin, eyes, hair, liver, gastrointestinal tract and brain function, and help support healthy heart function, enhance and stimulate the immune system and inhibit the growth of cancerous cells and tumours. They also help with Crohn's disease and anxiety, depression, fatigue, diabetes, epilepsy, canker sores, heart disease, infertility, multiple sclerosis, rosacea and psoriasis, amongst others. The B vitamins are also coenzymes involved in energy production. B-complex is important for elderly people and a deficiency can mimic Alzheimer's disease.

A team of American and Chinese researchers has discovered that Vitamin B9 (folic acid) is highly effective in preventing breast cancer in women. The researchers found a clear correlation between dietary intake of folic acid and the risk of breast cancer. It is also estimated that individuals with low vitamin B6 levels have a five times greater risk of having a heart attack than individuals with higher B6 levels.

Vitamin B-complex helps in the treatment of numerous health conditions, including ADHD and Alzheimer's disease.

The recommended dosage of vitamin B-complex is 50 mg a day.

Vitamin C

The famous two-time Nobel laureate Linus Pauling PhD spent years on research that has done much to reveal the powerful healing potential of vitamin C. He believed that as many as 75 per cent of all cancer deaths could be avoided through the proper use of this vitamin. Vitamin C is one of the most potent antioxidants known to science and is a powerful free radical scavenger. It protects against abnormal cells and prevents the destruction of DNA. It also stimulates the production of interferon, a powerful anti-cancer agent.

Vitamin C (also known as ascorbic acid) is found in every cell of our bodies and performs a multitude of functions: it assists in iron and calcium absorption, fights infection and plays an essential role in the health of the immune system. It reduces cholesterol and high blood pressure to help prevent arteriosclerosis. It is also vital for the growth and repair of body tissue cells, gums, blood vessels, teeth and bones. As for dosage, Dr Pauling recommended 10,000 mg a day. This may seem high but it is perfectly safe to take this high dose, as the body will naturally excrete any excess. Note though that if you do take a high dosage you will need to build up to it over the course of a week or two, as high doses can lead to diarrhoea, at least initially. If this does happen, reduce your dosage by half and then gradually build back up to taking higher levels.

The recommended dosage of vitamin C is 2,000–10,000 mg a day, but please be aware of the above cautions.

Vitamin D

Vitamin D is absorbed from sunlight and its deficiency has impacted on human health particularly in the past few hundred years. The advent of pollution since the Industrial Revolution has had an increasing effect of reducing vitamin D levels particularly for those living in developed urban areas. This has been exacerbated by the growing tendency for humans to spend more and more time indoors. Low levels of this vital vitamin can cause fragile bones, bent spines and weaken the muscles and can contribute to a myriad of health conditions such as osteoporosis, asthma, hypertension, heart disease and cancer.

A natural way to increase vitamin D levels is to make sure to get adequate direct sunlight. When your skin is exposed to sunlight you make vitamin D from the cholesterol in your skin. It is therefore recommended that you get direct sun exposure to your skin without the use of any sunscreen for 30 minutes a day. Because of the dangers of skin cancer it is recommended that you do this at times when the sun is not at its strongest, in the early morning or late afternoon.

In addition to direct sunlight it is advisable to take a vitamin D supplement and I suggest that you take 5000 IU per day. Because vitamin D can be stored in the body, I recommend that you monitor and adjust this based upon your actual vitamin D levels as indicated in your blood tests. Although the recommended daily allowance of vitamin D is 400 IU, more modern research has indicated that this is far too low.

The recommended daily dosage of vitamin D is 5000 IU a day.

Vitamin E

Vitamin E is a fat-soluble vitamin of critical importance in the prevention of a number of medical conditions including cancer, cardiovascular disease, diabetes, arthritis, cataracts and ageing. It is a potent antioxidant and has a powerful effect on the brain. Vitamin E also protects us against free radicals, causes dilation of the blood vessels – permitting a fuller flow of blood to the heart – and inhibits coagulation of the blood, preventing clots from forming.

Observational studies have associated lower rates of heart disease with higher vitamin E intake. A study of approximately 90,000 nurses suggested that the incidence of heart disease was 30 to 40 per cent lower in the nurses with the highest intake of vitamin E.

Vitamin E has been shown to fight cancer cells during radiation therapy without affecting normal cells. When combined with vitamin C and selenium, it helps to reduce the growth of breast and prostate cancer cells.

The recommended dosage of vitamin E is 1,000 mg a day.

Zinc

Zinc is an essential mineral and plays an important role in prostate gland function as well as in the growth and health of the reproductive organs. It is also required for the synthesis of protein and the formation of collagen, as well as playing an important part in promoting a healthy immune system, assisting in wound healing and being involved in the body's ability to taste and smell. Zinc also protects the liver from chemical damage and is vital for bone formation, as well as being a constituent of insulin and many other of the body's important enzymes.

Zinc also has powerful antioxidant qualities and an adequate intake is necessary to assist the body's use of vitamin E in the blood. Zinc also has synergy with many other vitamins, which means that it assists their absorption into the body.

The recommended dosage of zinc is 30 mg a day.

Chromium

The trace element chromium is vital for the body to function properly. The body stores chromium in the blood and the hair.

Chromium's principal role is as a Glucose Tolerant Factor (GTF). In other words, it is responsible for stimulating the activity of insulin in the body. When insulin is activated, it is able to assist in the process of metabolising sugars, which is how the body's tissues and cells obtain the energy they need to carry out activities such as muscle building and nervous system function. Insulin activity is also what helps people who are trying to lose weight; if glucose ends up being stored in the blood because the body isn't metabolising sugar properly, it can lead to a condition called insulin resistance. The excess glucose in the blood in this condition is stored as fat rather than burned as energy.

Chromium has other responsibilities too. It helps to control levels of cholesterol in the blood and also helps control fat levels. For these reasons, among others, chromium is currently being actively studied so that researchers can find out more about its role in reducing heart-related conditions.

The recommended dosage of chromium is 50 mg a day.

Selenium

Selenium is a nutrient that plays a critical role in the production of antioxidant enzymes that protect cells against the effects of free radicals that are produced during normal oxygen metabolism; it is essential for normal functioning of the immune system. The body develops defences such as selenium antioxidants to control levels of free radicals because they can damage cells and contribute to the development of some chronic diseases, such as BPH and prostate cancer.

This naturally occurring trace mineral protects your body against free radicals generated by smoke, pollution, radiation, and other environmental toxins. Selenium helps maintain healthy muscles and red blood cells. Selenium helps to regulate immune function and acts to detoxify the body of heavy metal toxins. It aids in the production of antibodies and helps maintain a healthy heart and liver and, when combined with vitamin E and zinc, helps provide relief from an enlarged prostate. Studies have shown some positive effects of selenium when used in the treatment of arthritis, cardio-vascular disease, male infertility, AIDS and high blood pressure. Further scientific studies have shown that selenium inhibits the growth of tumors, and there is some evidence that AIDS patients also have benefited when they take a selenium supplement as it increases red and white blood cell counts.

Its other benefits include being involved with iodine metabolism, pancreatic function, DNA repair, immunity and the detoxification of heavy metals.

The recommended dosage of selenium is 200 mcg a day.

Coenzyme Q10 (CoQ10)
Imagine that each and every cell in your body is a tiny engine. This engine uses oxygen to burn the fuels provided by food. CoQ10 is part of the engine that provides the 'spark' for this process. No other substance will substitute for CoQ10. Without CoQ10 there can be no spark and therefore no production of energy.

Research has demonstrated the health benefits of taking CoQ10; some of them are improved cardiovascular function and blood circulation, increased energy levels and less fatigue, lowered blood pressure and reduced angina. It may also help prevent or slow Alzheimer's and Parkinson's diseases, and is a strong antioxidant and anti-ageing agent. CoQ10 is found in all food but is easily destroyed by cooking, which means that most people don't get enough in their diet.

When it comes to cardiovascular benefits, it has been shown that people with poor heart muscle contraction benefit greatly from CoQ10, as it increases heart contraction strength and boosts health recovery. CoQ10 has also been shown to aid in the full or partial remission of breast tumours, as well as retarding tumour growth in general. There are over 300 published papers on the disease-preventing roles of CoQ10.

The recommended dosage of CoQ10 is 400 mg a day.

L-carnosine

L-carnosine is one of the most popular anti-ageing supplements recommended by anti-ageing specialists. It is a natural dipeptide consisting of the amino acids beta-alanine and L-histidine, and is naturally present in all the cells of the body.

L-carnosine levels are high in young people but start to decline with age, starting at around 40. Stress and trauma also seem to cause a reduction in levels.

The exact biological role of L-carnosine is not yet very well understood, but many studies indicate that it has strong anti-oxidant properties and, consequently, anti-ageing effects. Many animal studies indicate that it protects against radiation damage, improves heart function and promotes wound healing. There are also strong indications that L-carnosine plays other roles, including helping to clear the body of toxic heavy metals. In addition, it appears to act as a chemical messenger in the nervous system, helping to improve its function, and studies have shown that it can rejuvenate cells at the end of their lifecycle, thus restoring and extending their lifespan.

L-carnosine may also help to prevent and perhaps even treat age-related conditions, including neurological degeneration, the accumulation of damaged proteins and muscle atrophy.

The recommended dosage of L-carnosine is 500 mg a day.

MSM

MSM, or to give it its full name, methyl-sulfonyl-methane, is a natural form of organic sulphur that is present in low concentrations throughout the body's tissues. Many foods contain MSM but it is greatly depleted during the cooking process. MSM helps maintain healthy cells and is supportive of good immune function. It is a scavenger of free radicals and foreign proteins, and so cleans the bloodstream, helping with allergies to things like food and pollens.

You cannot overdose on MSM; your body will use what it needs and then flush out any excess. To maintain healthy cells, it is recommended that you take MSM every morning and evening.

The recommended dosage of MSM is 2,000 mg a day.

Live-Long Code Nutrition Plan Tips

Staying youthful and staying healthy go hand in hand. And staying healthy is governed, to a large degree, by your eating habits. If they have become just that – habits, with little or no thought put into them – it is quite likely that your diet doesn't have an ideal balance of nutrients and calories.

The following dietary guidelines will help you incorporate sound nutritional habits into your daily life. They are simple tips and are especially useful if you have not focused on a balanced diet before.

1. Be aware of the quantity of calories you need to maintain your Live-Long Code target weight.
2. Relax and sit comfortably when eating. Chew your food very thoroughly before swallowing. Remember the Chinese saying, 'drink your food and eat your drink'. Eat slowly, enjoying each mouthful. When you eat slowly you prepare your food more adequately for digestion; the food's cell walls are better broken down so that the vitamins, minerals and antioxidants can better be made available to our bodies. Another good reason to eat slowly is that it helps you adhere to calorie restriction; the more you chew, the more satisfied you will feel. You will also take longer to eat your meals, which will lessen your inclination to overeat.
3. Eat six small meals per day, rather than the traditional three square meals. In this way, you will maintain a balance in your blood sugar and the level of nutrients in your body throughout the day.
4. Choose quality over quantity. Shredding, dicing and thinly slicing food makes it easier to digest. Overeating is to be avoided as it puts a strain on digestion. It is usually recommended that you should eat only to the point where you are 80 per cent full.
5. There is a famous saying or proverb, 'Eat breakfast like a king, lunch like a prince and dinner like a pauper.' What this means

is that you should eat your larger meals earlier in the day. This gives your body a chance to burn the calories you've consumed, and, more importantly, means that while you are sleeping your body will be able to work on healing itself rather than trying to digest large amounts of food.

6. The best methods of cooking are stir-frying and steaming. Foods prepared by these methods cook quickly and therefore retain their vital nutrients better than if you slow-cook food.

7. Foods should generally be served at room temperature or warmer and eating straight from the fridge is discouraged. The body has to work to heat cold foods, which impairs the digestive process.

8. Main courses should be supplemented with green or jasmine tea, which are considered good aids to digestion.

The Live-Long Code Suggested Menus

Breakfast

Bircher Muesli
Berry Couscous
Mushrooms and Scrambled Eggs on Wholegrain Bread
Low-Fat Banana and Raspberry Smoothie
Carrot and Mushroom Stir-Fry

Lunch

Ambrosia Salad
Baked Mushrooms Contra Costa
Chicken and Sweetcorn Soup
Spiced Pumpkin and Lentil Soup
Chicken and Mango Salad with Honey Dressing
Bamboo-steamed Fish and Vegetables
Ratatouille
Green tea after lunch

Dinner

Zesty Grilled Turkey Breast
Ginger Tofu Slices
Fennel Salmon
Stuffed Trout
Spicy Lemon Broccoli
Mexican Salad with Chicken
Green tea after dinner

Dessert

Pear and Banana Ambrosia
Fresh Cinnamon Apple Sauce
Marinated Strawberries

Snack Options

Fresh fruit
Dried fruit
Nut mix (unsalted)

For further menu options, please consult www.immortalitycode.com.

Breakfast Recipes

Bircher Muesli

Serves 8

2 cups rolled oats
1 cup muesli
2 cups hot water
2 tbsp lemon juice
¼ cup almonds
200 g low-fat organic yoghurt
1 large apple, grated

The Live-Long Code

2 tbsp honey
150 g fruit (berries, peaches and bananas)

Put the oats and muesli in a large dish and pour over the water and lemon juice. Soak for half an hour. Add the almonds, yoghurt and apple and mix thoroughly. Cover and place in the refrigerator overnight. While serving, add the honey and fruit. This muesli will keep for four days.

Berry Couscous

Serves 4

1 cup couscous
1 cup apple and 1 cup blackcurrant juice
1 cinnamon stick
2 cups raspberries
2 cups blueberries
2 cups halved strawberries
2 tsp lemon zest
1 tbsp shredded mint
200 g low-fat organic yoghurt
2 tbsp honey

Place the couscous in a bowl. Pour the juice into a saucepan and add the cinnamon stick. Boil and pour over the couscous. Cover the bowl and leave to stand for around 5 minutes, until the liquid is absorbed. Remove the cinnamon stick and refrigerate.

Mix the couscous grains and add the berries, lemon zest and mint. Pour the mixture into four bowls. Serve with yoghurt and honey.

Mushrooms with Scrambled Eggs and Wholegrain Bread

Serves 4

8 mushrooms
2 tomatoes, halved

extra virgin olive oil
3 tbsp balsamic vinegar
4 eggs, lightly beaten
2 tbsp fresh chopped chives
3 tbsp skimmed milk
8 slices wholegrain bread

Slice the mushrooms and put them in a baking tray with the tomatoes. Lightly drizzle with extra virgin olive oil. Sprinkle with balsamic vinegar and season with freshly ground pepper. Bake for 10 to 15 minutes, until tender.

Put the eggs, chives and milk in a bowl and stir together. Pour the mixture into a wok and cook for 2–3 minutes, stirring gently with a wooden spoon to scramble.

Serve the scrambled eggs on the wholegrain bread along with the mushrooms and tomato.

Low-Fat Banana and Raspberry Smoothie

Serves 4

3 cups skimmed milk
2 bananas
1 cup raspberries
1 tbsp oat bran
1 cup low-fat organic yoghurt

Pour the milk into a covered container and place in the freezer for half an hour. Chop the bananas and put them in a blender. Add the raspberries, oat bran and yoghurt and half of the milk. Blend for around 30 seconds, until smooth.

Pour in the remaining milk and blend for another 30 seconds, until all the ingredients are combined. Pour into four glasses and serve immediately.

Carrot and Mushroom Stir-Fry

Serves 4

6 carrots, sliced
4 tsp extra virgin olive oil
5 spring onions, sliced
10 mushrooms, sliced
½ tsp black pepper
juice from half a lemon

Steam the carrots until tender. Heat the oil in a wok. Add the carrots, spring onions and mushrooms and stir-fry until cooked. Mix in the lemon juice and pepper and serve.

Lunch Recipes

Ambrosia Salad

Serves 4

6 carrots, shredded
¼ cup walnuts
2 cups diced pineapple
1 tbsp lemon juice
¼ cup raisins

Mix all the ingredients in a large bowl. Cover and chill in the refrigerator before serving.

Baked Mushrooms Contra Costa

Serves 4

12 large mushrooms
4 tbsp lemon juice
2 tbsp extra virgin olive oil
2 tbsp fresh chopped parsley

1 clove garlic
2 tbsp minced onion
1 tsp black pepper
3 tbsp dry sherry

Place the mushroom caps on a baking tray and sprinkle with the lemon juice. Mince the mushroom stems and sauté in the extra virgin olive oil. Mix the sautéed mushroom stems with the remaining ingredients to make stuffing. Pour the stuffing into the mushroom caps. Cover and bake at 175°C/350°F for 15 minutes.

Chicken and Sweetcorn Soup

Serves 4

1 tbsp extra virgin olive oil
1 onion, finely chopped
1 celery stick, diced
1 garlic clove, crushed
2 tsp grated ginger
2 cooked corn cobs, kernels removed
1 litre reduced-salt chicken stock
¼ cup soy sauce
500 g chicken mince
4 spring onions, finely sliced
¼ cup chopped fresh coriander

Heat the oil in a saucepan. Add the onion, celery, garlic and ginger and cook for 4 minutes, until soft. Add the corn and chicken stock and bring to the boil. Reduce the heat and simmer for 10 minutes. Remove from the heat and allow to cool.

Transfer the ingredients to a blender and mix, leaving the soup slightly chunky. Bring to the boil and simmer for a further 10 minutes.

Spiced Pumpkin and Lentil Soup

Serves 4

1 tbsp extra virgin olive oil
1 onion, chopped
3 garlic cloves, chopped
1 tsp ground turmeric
½ tsp ground cumin
½ tsp ground coriander
½ tsp chilli flakes
5 cups chopped pumpkin
½ cup red lentils
4 cups water

Heat the oil in a saucepan. Add the onion and garlic and fry for 5 minutes, until softened. Add the turmeric, cumin, coriander and chilli flakes and fry for a further 2 minutes. Add the pumpkin, red lentils and 4 cups of boiling water. Bring to the boil, then reduce the heat and simmer. Cover for approximately 20 minutes, until the pumpkin and lentils are tender. Cool for 5 minutes.

Pour the contents into a blender and mix for 30 seconds, until evenly chopped. Season well with ground black pepper and reheat.

Chicken and Mango Salad with Honey Dressing

Serves 4

2 tbsp vinegar
3 tsp honey
3 cm piece of ginger, chopped
1 tbsp canola oil
1 tsp sesame oil
125g salad leaves
1 large mango, thinly sliced
½ red onion, sliced

1 cup halved cherry tomatoes
1 cup mangetout
4 cooked chicken breasts, shredded

Put the vinegar, honey and ginger in a blender and process for 20 seconds, until finely chopped. Slowly pour in the oils and blend for a further 20 seconds, until you have made a thick and creamy dressing. Arrange the salad leaves on the serving plates and top with the mango, onion, tomatoes, mangetout and chicken. Drizzle with the dressing and serve immediately.

Bamboo-Steamed Fish and Vegetables

Serves 4

4 large lettuce leaves
4 red snapper fillets
2 tbsp chopped fresh dill
pinch of black pepper
1 lemon, thinly sliced into 8 slices
4 cups broccoli florets
30 cherry tomatoes
mixed herbs

Line the lower tier of a bamboo steamer with the lettuce leaves. Place a fish fillet on top of each leaf. Sprinkle with the dill and pepper and place two lemon slices on each fillet. Place the broccoli and tomatoes in the upper tier of the steamer and sprinkle with the mixed herbs. Place the upper steamer on the lower tier and cover with the lid.

Pour 2 inches of water into a pan that fits the steamer. Place the steamer on the pan and bring the water to the boil. Make sure that the water never touches the bottom of the steamer. Steam for 15 minutes, until the fish flakes easily. Serve immediately.

Ratatouille

Serves 4

1 large onion, chopped
1 clove garlic, minced
2 tbsp extra virgin olive oil
½ lb aubergine, diced
½ lb courgette, sliced
2 large tomatoes, skinned and wedged
1 green pepper, sliced and seeded
1 tbsp chopped fresh parsley
½ tsp oregano
pinch of black pepper

Sauté the onion and garlic in the extra virgin olive oil until tender. Pour in the remaining ingredients and bring to the boil. Reduce the heat, cover and let simmer for half an hour, until the vegetables are tender.

Dinner Recipes

Zesty Grilled Turkey Breast

Serves 4

4 garlic cloves, *minced*
½ cup lemon juice
¼ cup flaxseed oil
1 tsp paprika
1 tsp cumin
1 tsp turmeric
½ tsp white pepper
700 g turkey breast slices
1 tbsp extra virgin olive oil

Put all the ingredients except the turkey and olive oil into a blender and mix for 20 seconds. Drizzle the turkey breasts with the extra virgin olive oil and grill for 5 minutes on each side. Top each breast with 3 tablespoons of the sauce and serve.

Ginger Tofu Slices

Serves 4

500 g tofu
1 tbsp of grated ginger
2 tbsp of soy sauce
2 tsp of sesame oil
2 tbsp of mirin
½ tbsp extra virgin olive oil
2 tbsp of finely chopped spring onions

Cut the tofu into eight thin slices and drain on paper towels while you prepare the marinade. Squeeze the grated ginger to get approximately 2 teaspoons of ginger juice. Mix the ginger juice, soy sauce, sesame oil and mirin together to make a marinade. Place the tofu slices in a shallow bowl and pour the marinade over. Marinate the tofu on both sides for a total of 20 minutes. Remove the tofu and allow it to drain for a minute to remove excess salt from the marinade. Heat the extra virgin olive oil in a wok and fry the tofu on one side for 2 to 3 minutes until it is golden brown. Flip the slices over and fry for another 2 minutes. Remove, place on a serving plate and garnish with the finely chopped spring onions and salad.

Fennel Salmon

Serves 4

3 tbsp extra virgin olive oil
1 bulb fresh fennel, cored and thinly sliced
700 g salmon fillets
1 tsp dried basil
1 tsp dried dill
2 cups broccoli, steamed

The Live-Long Code

Preheat the oven to 200°C/400°F. Coat the bottom of a glass baking tray with 2 tablespoons of extra virgin olive oil. Place the fennel at the bottom of the dish and layer the salmon over the top. Drizzle the rest of the olive oil over the top and sprinkle with the basil and dill. Bake for 20 minutes and serve with steamed broccoli.

Stuffed Trout

Serves 4

½ tsp dried dill
2 tbsp finely chopped, parsley
2 tbsp finely chopped onion
¼ cup sliced almonds
500 g trout
juice of 1 lemon
½ tsp ground black pepper

Preheat the oven to 200°C/400°F. Mix the dill, parsley, onion and almonds in a bowl and fill the trout with the mixture. Place the fish on foil and pour over the lemon juice. Add the pepper and seal the foil over the trout. Bake for 25 minutes, until the fish flakes easily.

Spicy Lemon Broccoli

Serves 4

4 cups broccoli florets
1 tbsp extra virgin olive oil
2 tsp freshly grated lemon peel
crushed red pepper to taste

Place a steamer on a saucepan and fill the pan with water to just below the steamer. Place the broccoli in the steamer and bring to the boil. Cover and cook for 3 minutes. Remove the broccoli. Heat the extra virgin olive oil in a wok over a medium heat. Add the lemon peel and crushed red pepper to taste. Stir-fry for about 1 minute, until the peel starts to brown. Add the broccoli and stir-fry for a further minute. Serve immediately.

Mexican Salad with Chicken

Serves 4

6 cups chopped lettuce
8 spring onions, thinly sliced
24 cherry tomatoes, halved
6 tbsp extra virgin olive oil
450 g chicken
½ cup diced green chillies
½ cup water
2 tbsp garlic powder
2 tbsp onion powder
2 tsp dry mustard
2 tsp cayenne pepper
2 ripe avocados, thinly sliced

Place the lettuce, spring onions and tomatoes on two large plates and set aside. Heat the extra virgin olive oil over a low heat in a wok. Add the chicken and remaining ingredients apart from the avocado and simmer for 15 minutes, stirring throughout. Remove from the heat and place on each salad. Place the avocado slices on top and serve immediately.

Dessert Recipes

Pear and Banana Ambrosia

Serves 4

2 pears, cored and peeled
2 ripe avocados
2 bananas
1 cup lemon juice

The Live-Long Code

1 mango, peeled and sliced
1 cup crushed ice

Put all the ingredients in a blender and mix until smooth. Put in the freezer for 10 minutes and serve cold.

Fresh Cinnamon Apple Sauce

Serves 4

12 apples
5 tbsp fresh lemon juice
2 tsp cinnamon

Peel, core and slice the apples. Place in a blender with the lemon juice and mix until smooth. Sprinkle with cinnamon and serve.

Marinated Strawberries

Serves 4

1 litre strawberries, washed and halved
juice of 4 lemons
1 tsp honey
1 tbsp balsamic vinegar

Mix the strawberries and lemon juice in a large bowl. Stir and refrigerate for 2 hours. When you're ready to serve, mix the honey and balsamic vinegar and drizzle over the strawberries.

Preparing and Eating Your Food

It's vital to eat the right food, but it's also important to eat in the correct way. The following approaches are recommended as part of your Live-Long Code guide to healthy eating.

- Variety is encouraged and you should avoid consuming too much of the same foods at the expense of others.

- There should be strong emphasis on eating fresh organic food where possible.
- Always make sure you wash fruit and vegetables thoroughly, as they may have been exposed to chemical pesticides.
- Ingredients should be shredded, diced or thinly sliced; this makes them easier to digest.
- Foods should generally be served at room temperature or warmer; you should try to avoid eating food direct from the fridge. Your body has to expend energy heating cold food, which impairs the digestive process.
- Overeating is discouraged as it puts a strain on digestion. It is better to eat smaller portions frequently throughout the day than fewer larger meals.
- Breakfast should be considered the most important meal of the day, and ideally all or most of your food should be consumed before 6 p.m. This gives your body a chance to burn off the calories from the food and means that while you're sleeping your body is repairing itself rather than spending energy digesting food.
- Always relax and sit comfortably when eating; it aids digestion.

Summary

- Adopting the correct eating habits is a proven way to extend lifespan. By adopting the Live-Long Code Nutrition Plan in its entirety you optimise your chances of success. If you can, make the changes to your diet quickly and completely; this approach delivers benefits and success far more quickly.
- Be aware of good and bad cholesterol and combine fruit, vegetables, whole grains and healthier white meats. Avoid dairy, salt, saturated and trans fats and all refined carbohydrates.
- While supplements should never replace healthy nutrition, there are benefits to taking certain mineral and vitamin supplements, especially when you are following a calorie restriction diet.

The Live-Long Code Nutrition Plan identifies which food elements are optimal for longevity. But what can you do to help you implement the plan as effectively as possible? What other environmental and lifestyle choices should you make to enhance your life-extending potential? The Live-Long Code Nutrition Plan looks at what is best to put into your body. Next we look at what toxic elements you should seek to avoid and remove from your body – the Live-Long Code Detox.

CHAPTER FIVE

The Live-Long Code Detox

Removing toxins from your body is one of the most effective ways to rejuvenate your health for prolonged life. I spend a considerable amount of time with my clients discussing what burdens they are placing on their bodies because of toxic elements. It is worth examining all the potential factors that could mean that you are overloading your body with toxins, so that you can then eliminate as many as possible from your life to decrease the toxic burden on your body. Your organs will then be less stressed, improving their capacity to function and consequently improving your health. Decreasing the toxins in your body also means that you lessen your chances of developing disease and illness in the first place.

There are many harmful elements that could be hindering our health. Some of these come from the environment, both indoor and outdoor, some come from what we eat, drink or use on our bodies and others are associated with behavioural choices. One element may not be too damaging in itself, but the cumulative effect of all of these toxins acting continuously upon our bodies can often be very detrimental. We each get compromised in different ways, possibly due to genetic predisposition – for example, one person might develop an allergic reaction or sensitivity, another could develop a heart condition and a third might develop cancer. Eastern medicine recognises the importance of removing or at least reducing these factors before you start to make other changes.

Decreasing your toxic exposure and load takes time and awareness, not to mention commitment. In this chapter we will look at decreasing your toxic load and strategies for how best to achieve this. Depending on your personal level of toxic exposure, this part of the Live-Long Code will vary from individual to individual. Whatever your personal load, though, make step-by-step changes in habits and behavioural patterns and in a relatively short space of time you will have made changes that will dramatically enhance your well being.

Reducing Toxic Exposure

Before you go about starting to remove toxins from your body, you need to look at reducing your existing exposure to toxins. As mentioned, each individual might respond to environmental toxins in different ways, and most of us can tolerate these toxins for many years without any obvious repercussions. However, over time toxic load increases, and at some point we might find ourselves adversely affected, seemingly suddenly and out of nowhere. How can this happen? It seems reasonable to imagine that things that are harmful to us would be immediately evident. But despite the fact that the world around us is awash with chemicals, many of these toxins cannot be seen, smelled, tasted or felt. Because our bodies are designed for survival, we develop a tolerance for these substances. However, just because we have some tolerance does not mean that these toxins are not detrimental to us; they are, particularly when they accumulate.

Are You Toxic?

Toxicity is one of the biggest strains on our health. Our world is polluted to the point that there are genuine and serious concerns about the long-term viability of the planet, and in particular of our survival as a species. To survive we all need air to breathe, clean water that we can safely drink and nutritious food that we can safely eat.

Ask yourself the following questions, they will help you to determine if you might have a high level of toxicity in your body.

- Are you sensitive to skin creams and odours?
- Have you become increasingly intolerant towards certain foods and drinks?
- Have you recently noticed a stronger reaction to caffeine or alcohol?
- Do you suffer from any autoimmune conditions?
- Do you have skin problems such as acne, eczema, dermatitis or itchy skin?
- Do you suffer from fatigue, joint pain, unusual or unexplained muscular pain or weakness?
- Are you subject to fluctuations in your mental state or depression?
- Do you get headaches?
- Do you suffer with sinus problems?
- Do you catch colds frequently?
- Do you drink more than two alcoholic drinks on an average day?
- Do you use drugs – prescription or otherwise – on a regular basis?

The chances are that most of us will answer yes to one or more of the above questions, which means that most of us would do well to try to reduce our exposure to toxins. Of course there are some things we cannot change overnight. For example, it would be a mistake to stop taking prescription drugs without the approval and supervision of your doctor. However, there are some toxic elements that you can eliminate safely.

Potential Toxins

- Outdoor industrial and traffic pollution.
- Indoor pollution from:
    - carpets
    - dust
    - household cleaning products
    - household chemicals such as paint
    - chemicals in water and food
    - processed food

- food colourings, preservatives, additives and flavourings
- chemical pesticides
- food packaging
- personal-care products
- heavy metal exposure (e.g. mercury in dental amalgam)
- radiation
- drugs
  - prescriptions
  - recreational
  - legal (e.g. alcohol, tobacco)
- allergies
  - pollen
  - dust mites
- diet
  - trans fats
  - refined carbohydrates.

The wear and tear theory of ageing believes that the effects of ageing are caused by damage done to cells and body systems over time. Essentially, these systems 'wear out' due to use and exposure to radiation, toxins and ultraviolet light, which can damage our genes. The effects of our body's own functioning can also cause damage. When the body metabolises oxygen, free radicals are produced that can cause damage to cells and tissues, and once these cells and tissues wear out, they can no longer function correctly. The Live-Long Code Detox Programme addresses this issue and works on the following principles.

1. A primary cause of illness is the accumulation of unnecessary waste, resulting in toxic accumulation, poison retention and subsequently disease.
2. Your body is designed to support optimal function and gives a variety of signals (including illness) when there are toxins in your body.

3. Given the proper environment and the removal of these toxins, your body has the power to both stay healthy and repair previous harm done, returning it to a normal healthy state.

The pattern of disease over the past 100 years has changed. Diseases such as measles and tuberculosis used to be a huge threat, but now, due to improved standards of living in the developed world and advances in medicine, these diseases are much more under control. Today's 'new' illnesses and the increased incidence of illnesses such as heart disease, diabetes, cancer, chronic fatigue and MS, as well as asthma and allergies, have paralleled human beings' increased exposure to modern toxins.

The toxin levels in our environment are higher now than ever before in human history, and despite efforts to bring this pattern to a halt the signs are that this will continue to increase. Without necessarily knowing it, we have all to some degree been contaminated and poisoned by toxic chemicals. Our bodies were not designed to encounter such a heavy onslaught, and as a result of their inability to break down these chemicals, the toxins build up and play havoc with our organ systems. The consequence of this toxic poisoning has been the escalating volume of the illnesses listed above.

Of course, we can't completely avoid exposure to toxic chemicals; the simple act of living puts us in direct contact with harmful materials. When we eat foods that have been exposed to pesticides, additives and pollutants, we are allowing toxic substances into our body. Even with organic food, there will still have been some pollution in the soil and air the food grew in. Our skin is also exposed to chemicals in cosmetics, detergents and toiletries. The air that we breathe is contaminated by car fumes, industrial waste and environmental pollutants.

It is hard to say to exactly what point illnesses are related to toxic exposure. We all have a different genetic make-up and live in different environments, which makes it difficult for scientists to identify direct links between the many illnesses that exist and people's exposure to the wide variety of toxic chemicals in existence. Nevertheless, the increased incidence of 'modern' illnesses and the parallel increase in exposure to toxic chemicals suggest that limiting our toxic exposure and eliminating toxins as best we can should be a component of the Live-Long Code Programme.

The dietary approach taken in our nutrition plan is also the optimum approach to combating the toxins present in food and drink. That is to say that by implementing this nutrition plan you are almost halfway there. Let's therefore focus first on ways to approach implementing the nutrition plan.

The Live-Long Code Kitchen Clearout

As a first step to adopting the Live-Long Code Nutrition Plan, I highly recommend that you remove all the unhealthy foods from your kitchen. Out of sight means out of mind! Of course if all members of your household want to be healthier and to live longer, the entire household will want to adopt the Live-Long Code Nutrition Plan and you can then do a full kitchen clearout. If, however, only some members of the household want to follow the plan, you need to identify cupboard, fridge and kitchen space that is dedicated to those people who will be implementing the plan. Give yourself plenty of time to do this, as you may have to examine items one by one and look carefully at the ingredients list. To begin the kitchen clearout, remove the following foods from your kitchen space:

- All canned food.
- All processed food.
- Anything containing MSG, artificial sweeteners, preservatives, flavourings and colourings.
- Beer.
- Biscuits.
- Breakfast cereals.
- Butter.
- Cakes.
- Cheeses.
- Chocolate.
- Coffee.

- Crisps.
- Dairy milk.
- Non-free-range eggs.
- Ice cream.
- Jam and marmalade.
- Margarine containing hydrogenated oil or trans fats.
- Popcorn.
- Processed white meat.
- Red meat and pork.
- Salt.
- Salted nuts.
- Soft drinks.
- Sugar.
- Sweets.
- White bread.
- White flour.
- Yoghurt.

Detoxing Your Cooking Utensils and Storage

Once you have removed the more harmful foods, it makes good sense to continue your clearout by removing utensils and other items that when used in preparing food can lead to toxic contamination.

It is best to avoid all plastic-based packaging such as cling-film and plastic wrap. These plastics contain carcinogenic substances that can easily get transferred to the food they are used to wrap. We now understand that the toxins found in plastic can also have hormone-mimicking properties; there is a suggestion that these could be linked to the rise in reproductive cancers. Rather than wrapping fruit, vegetables and fish in plastic, use paper packageing.

The best materials for cooking with are glass, wood, porcelain and earthenware. Non-stick cooking vessels can emit toxins from their synthetic lining. Aluminium pots and pans also increase toxic discharge. Stainless steel is fine for knives and forks.

Detoxing Your Cooking Approach

The best methods of cooking are stir-frying and steaming, as they ensure the retention of vital nutrients and vitamins.

Stir-Frying

Stir-frying, originally associated with Eastern cooking, is one of the healthiest ways to cook and is an easy and quick method for cooking white meat, fish and vegetables. Stir-frying is done fast, over a high heat, with just a minimum amount of extra virgin olive oil; the food is moved rapidly and constantly around the pan or wok to enable an equal distribution of heat. A sauce can be added at the end of the cooking process, with the ingredients allowed to steam in it briefly.

Because of the speed of stir-frying there is a minimum amount of vitamin loss from the food. The colour and texture of the food are also preserved, which makes the food more appealing to the eye. Typical stir-fry dishes contain just a small amount of meat or fish and relatively large quantities of vegetables, which is in line with the Live-Long Code Nutrition Plan guidelines.

If you don't already have one, I would suggest that you purchase a wok, which is a large, round-sloped pan. Because of their shape, woks enable the ingredients to fall to the bottom of the pan, where the heat is the most intense. The classic round-bottom wok is designed for cooking over a flame, but flat-bottomed versions are available for use on modern hobs.

Because you will be cooking very fast, it is important to prepare the ingredients prior to doing your stir-frying. This includes having the correct amounts of sauces and seasonings to hand. You should cut vegetables into small pieces to enable fast and even cooking. In Chinese medicine smaller pieces of food are also considered to be easier to digest. Larger vegetables such as carrots are usually cut into strips or thinly sliced, round vegetables are cut into pieces and broccoli and cauliflower are broken into small florets. It is good to cut vegetables at an angle, as this exposes more of their surface area and so it cooks more quickly. Fish and poultry are usually diced or cut into thin strips or wafer-thin slices; again, this facilitates fast cooking. Poultry, fish and tofu can be marinated for a few hours beforehand, as this helps to tenderise them as well as adding flavour.

When you have all your ingredients ready, you can begin cooking. Start by heating the wok and lightly drizzling extra virgin olive oil around the edge. This oil will quickly heat up and coat the inside and bottom of the heated wok. When the wok is very hot you can start adding the ingredients. It is usual to add the flavouring ingredients, such as ginger or garlic, first; they will flavour the oil, which will then transfer the flavours to the food. Then add the poultry, fish or thicker vegetables – whatever you are cooking that needs the longest time. Then add the remaining ingredients, obviously adding those that need the least amount of time last. Toss and stir the ingredients with a wooden spatula throughout the cooking process, or just gently shake the wok so the food keeps moving around. Adding sauce is usually the final step in the cooking process; once your sauce has thickened the dish is ready to be served.

Steaming

Steaming is another cooking method which has long been associated with Eastern cooking. It is one of the oldest cooking methods known, although it has had a surge in popularity in recent years. It is thought that steaming may even predate the discovery of fire, as it is believed that early man may have used the stones from hot springs to cook food.

Steaming involves cooking food in the steam produced by boiling water. In the East a bamboo steamer is often used – these are now available in the West, but the more usual Western method is to use a metal, perforated basket placed over a saucepan. If you do have a bamboo steamer you can use it over a wok. There are many other steamers available; special electrical steaming appliances, tiered pans with several steaming baskets, and petal steamers that open up to fit most saucepans and fold away for easy storage.

Steaming is a light and very healthy cooking method because no fat or oil whatsoever is added. Mineral and vitamin loss is also minimal, so valuable nutrients are preserved. Just as in stir-frying, the full colours, flavours and textures of the food are also retained, making the food pleasing to both the eye and the palate. Steaming also ensures that poultry and fish remain extremely tender.

To steam food:

- Position the steamer on a saucepan of boiling water and fit the lid on tightly so that the steam cannot escape. When you have allowed steam to build up, add the ingredients to the basket.
- Make sure that the steamer basket isn't touching the water or else the food will be boiled rather than steamed.
- You can line the steamer with a muslin cloth to prevent delicate food from breaking up.
- Don't allow the pan to boil dry. You can keep a separate pot of boiling water close to hand if you need to replenish the water in the saucepan.
- Steaming doesn't add flavour, so if you wish you can marinade the food in advance, season it after cooking or serve it with a sauce.
- Serve the vegetables from the steamer as soon as the cooking time is up. If they are allowed to remain in the steamer they will continue to cook even after the heat is turned off; vegetables will go soggy, break apart and discolour.

There are other cooking methods, but they are less healthy than stir-frying and steaming; I would suggest that these two methods should dominate your cooking. In particular you should avoid any method that requires you to use large amounts of oil or fat. Try to avoid overcooking as this has the potential to rob your food of vital minerals and vitamins. There are two cooking methods that I believe are particularly unhealthy; as such, they deserve special mention.

Microwaving

Microwave cooking robs your food and hence your body of vital nutrients and as such it should be avoided. Microwave cooking is a relatively new form of cooking and can hardly be described as natural. Microwaves can now be found in most homes, unfortunately. I say unfortunately because not only does food cooked in a microwave taste – in my opinion – not quite right, but it is proven to deplete the nutritional value of the food. More importantly, microwaves also pose a risk to long-term health.

How Do Microwaves Cook Food?

As discussed earlier in this chapter, there are many possible explanations for the increasing incidence of a variety of health conditions in the Western world: demineralised soils, environmental toxins, poor nutrition, processed foods – the list goes on. The microwave oven may well play a significant role too.

There is growing evidence of the risks posed to human health from the microwaves that are emitted by mobile phones and phone masts. These waves disrupt the cells in your body because of their electromagnetic field (EMF) frequencies. This also happens to your food when you cook it in a microwave. We are advised not to eat food straight from a microwave because the food continues to cook in your body.

When food is cooked by other methods, heat moves from outside to inside the food. With microwave cooking the reverse happens; food is cooked from within and a process takes place that can alter its chemical structure. The microwaves that the food is bombarded with cause molecules to rotate millions of times a second. The structure of these molecules is literally deformed by this process and new, unnatural compounds are created. These compounds can be difficult for your body to deal with. In addition, vitamins, minerals and proteins are damaged and food can lose its bioavailability – which means that you will be less able to absorb nutrients from it.

The Risks of Microwaves

Research is dreadfully lacking in this important area; however, below are the details of some very pertinent research.

Microwave technology was developed by the Germans during the Second World War as a radar system. Soldiers who gathered around these radars to warm themselves up developed illnesses, including cancer. It was the ability of microwaves to heat that led to Humboldt University in Berlin developing the technology to cook hot meals for soldiers fighting in the Soviet Union. However, just like the soldiers who had huddled around the radars, these soldiers also developed major problems with their immune systems. The use of microwaves in this way was subsequently banned.

In more recent times, a Swiss food scientist, Hans Hertel, conducted a small, carefully controlled study on microwave ovens in 1992. The participants in the study consumed microwaved food and then had their blood evaluated. The blood tests revealed that consumption of microwaved foods decreased haemoglobin values, white blood cells showed a short-term decrease and HDL (good cholesterol) declined.

There is also the suggestion that microwaves add potentially harmful toxins to your body because they absorb toxins from the packaging the food comes in. There is also the danger of exposure to harmful electromagnetic radiation from the microwave itself. If you have a microwave, my advice is to stop using it, or better still throw it out.

Barbecues

There are numerous health issues surrounding barbecuing food. First of all, there is the potentially carcinogenic smoke, containing benzopyrene, that is produced when you grill meat over charcoal. Then there are heterocyclic amines (HCAs), which are formed when meats are cooked at very high temperatures until they char. There is evidence indicating that HCAs are carcinogenic; for example, researchers from the National Cancer Institute in the United States have identified a link between the risk of stomach cancer and meats cooked until charred. There is also evidence that a high intake of barbecued meat is associated with an increased risk of developing colorectal, pancreatic and breast cancer; a German study revealed that women who frequently ate barbecued food had double the risk of developing breast cancer as compared to women who never eat barbecued food.

The high temperatures involved in barbecuing can cause biochemical mutations in the food, particularly when it has been cooked to the point of charring.

Putting it simply, you should avoid eating barbecued food.

Going Organic

The amount of chemicals and pesticides used in crop production is, in my opinion, shocking. The residues from these pesticides are found in our food and have been associated with many illnesses. No matter how well you wash food, residues will have seeped in. A step you can take to reducing your exposure to pesticides is to eat organic foods wherever possible. All non-organic fruit should be washed thoroughly, or the skins should be removed to avoid the residues.

As well as helping to eliminate pesticide residues from your body, organic food has been shown in studies to generally contain higher levels of vitamins and minerals.

Organic foods are increasingly easy to find, and with increased demand for them the price has become more reasonable too. It might well be worth paying that small amount more for good-quality food that is far more beneficial to your health.

Dental Detox

We all know that smoking, obesity and high cholesterol are the most common offenders when it comes to heart attacks and strokes, but research shows that neglected gums and teeth – poor dental hygiene – can be added to the list of things that increase your risk.

Bacterial infections are an independent risk factor for heart diseases, so if you are generally fit and healthy but not looking after your teeth, you're increasing your chances of getting heart disease. There are up to 700 different bacteria in the human mouth; most are benign, and some are important for good health, but a few can trigger a biological cascade leading to diseases of the arteries that are linked to heart attacks and stroke. Failing to brush your teeth helps those germs to flourish.

The mouth is probably the most polluted and toxic place in the human body, so if you have an open blood vessel from bleeding gums, bacteria and germs can gain entry into your bloodstream. Once inside the blood, certain bacteria stick to platelets, causing them to clot inside the vessel and thus reducing blood flow to the heart. This not only creates a condition that can provoke a heart attack and strokes, it also affects the immune system.

Maintaining good dental hygiene is therefore an essential part of the Live-Long Code Detox Programme. You should brush your teeth after every meal, plus in the morning and before you go to bed. A daily routine of brushing and flossing your teeth, together with regular dental checkups, is enough to prevent tooth decay and gum disease.

The Dangers of Amalgam

It's true that most dentists will tell you that amalgam fillings are harmless, but there is now a body of scientific research that suggests a different reality. Amalgam fillings contain mercury, which in all its forms is toxic; there is no level that is safe for your body. Prominent researcher Dr Boyd Haley, from the University of Kentucky, points out:

'We can't go inside a living human being and look at their brain, so we have to work outside, and do scientific experiments such as we've done. And to the best that we can determine with these experiments, mercury is a time-bomb in the brain, waiting to have an effect. If it's not bothering someone when they're young, especially when they age it can turn into something quite disastrous.'

The mercury used in dental amalgam is fully bioavailable – in other words it will be absorbed by your system. Mercury from amalgam fillings has been shown to be neurotoxic and capable of causing immune dysfunction and autoimmune diseases.

Amalgam fillings have been in use for about 180 years; they originated England and spread to Europe and America. They met with immediate acceptance by dentists because they provided a cheap and reasonably effective alternative to other filling techniques. However, it is generally accepted now, even by dentists, that someone trying to introduce legal amalgam now, would not be granted legal approval for use because of the serious questions that remain about its safety.

What Dentists Are Taught About Amalgam

Dentists are given very specific training in how to handle dental amalgam safely.

- Do not touch amalgam with bare hands: the mercury can enter the body through the skin.
- Use thorough ventilation: the mercury vapour produced from amalgam is easily absorbed into the body by inhalation.
- Amalgam cut out of teeth and left over from filling the teeth must be stored under photographic fixer in a sealed glass container. The high sulphur content of the solution helps to prevent the release of mercury vapour into the atmosphere.
- It is illegal to dispose of waste amalgam into sewerage or drain water: it will pollute the environment.
- Specialists in this field must dispose of waste amalgam as toxic waste.
- Mercury spills must be cleaned up immediately and must not be vacuumed: this will vaporise the mercury.

Therefore the only safe and legal place to keep this toxic waste is in the mouth of a living person! This is just crazy.

How Much Mercury Comes Out of Amalgam?

Mercury escapes from amalgam all the time. Increases in temperature, friction and electrical currents all cause an increase in the release of mercury vapour from amalgam throughout the life of the filling. Each time you have a hot drink, chew or grind your teeth, the levels of mercury coming from the amalgam will be elevated. This elevated level persists for about 90 minutes. Thus most of us on a regular cycle of eating and tooth-grinding will be living with a pretty much permanently elevated level of mercury vapour in our mouths.

Mercury is a cumulative poison; it stays in your body and the levels are topped up continuously. This form of poisoning is called micromercurialism and the earliest symptoms are sub-clinical neurological – in other words, fatigue, headaches, forgetfulness, reduced short-term memory, poor concentration, shyness and timidity, confusion, rapid mood swings, unprovoked anger, depression and suicidal tendencies.

Amalgam and the Immune System

True allergy to amalgam is only one type of immune reaction. There are literally hundreds of scientific papers discussing the damaging effects mercury can have on the immune system. Mercury from amalgam may result in an increase in allergies, skin rashes and itching. Additionally, a depleted immune system creates an environment in the body for other diseases to develop. When mercury binds to proteins, the immune system sees them as foreign substances and attacks them, which may lead to a cascade of events potentially ending in autoimmune diseases.

Mercury binds strongly to selenium, the trace element needed for a wide variety of enzyme functions. The latest research indicates a direct relationship between reduced blood selenium levels and an increase in the rate of cancer. Although this has been published in the alternative medical journals for years, it is only now becoming known in the traditional medical journals. The selenium depletion that is potentially happening in our bodies is one of the reasons why selenium supplements are recommended by the Live-Long Code Nutrition Plan.

What You Should Do

After reading this you may feel concerned enough to rush to your dentist and demand that all of your amalgam fillings be replaced. If you do take this route, make sure you go to a dentist who specialises in replacing amalgam fillings; unless the correct precautions are taken, you may be exposed to extremely high levels of mercury, which has the potential to make you seriously ill. Protocols do exist for the safe removal of amalgam – they have been designed to maximise the benefit of this type of treatment for the patient. Removing amalgam fillings will obviously remove this source of mercury from your body, which is likely to be the greatest source, but do remember that there will still be mercury stored in your body that will take time to come out.

There are alternatives to amalgam. If your dentist still believes that the alternatives are not as good as amalgam, perhaps you could suggest that he or she read the published literature demonstrating that amalgam is in fact one of the worst mechanical restorative materials. Alternately, you could change dentists. Even if you decide not to have your amalgam removed, there are some dietary supplements that have been shown to be helpful either in removing mercury from the body or in starting to repair some of the damage it causes. Research released in 1996 says that the only thing known to take mercury out of the brain and across the blood-brain barrier is fresh coriander. Additionally, two of the Live-Long Code's nutrition supplements help remove mercury from your body – spirulina and selenium.

Conquering Food Cravings – The Revulsion Effect

Changing your diet is challenging. Foods that have been a central part of your diet for many years can often feel like part of who you are. When I changed my own diet I changed it completely, literally overnight; there are foods that had been a regular part of my diet that I have never eaten again. I did have food cravings; I felt pangs and cravings for sugar in the form of sweet food. Whenever this happened I would imagine the harmful bacteria and cells – the kind of things that had lived off this sugar – creating discomfort for me in an effort to force me to feed them sugar again, as they were beginning to starve. The harsher my cravings were, the closer I felt I was getting to victory over these harmful bacteria. This mental technique proved very effective. Making such a radical change in the food that you eat may seem difficult, but doing it this way is more effective than making partial changes. When your goals are vague or blurred your mind becomes less clear about what you are attempting to achieve; as a result you are more likely to fail. There are a number of powerful methods you can use to support rapid changes in your eating habits and make an effective transition to your new healthy eating regime. Perhaps the most powerful of these methods involves the use of mental revulsion.

Many substances that later become addictive are often not pleasant when you first experience them. For example, when people smoke for the first time they will almost invariably have an unpleasant experience. For many people this is enough to put them off for life – and lucky for them. Others persist despite this unpleasant experience until they have forced themselves into accepting the habit. Through persistence and mental conditioning people manage to train their bodies to accept bad and poisonous habits.

The revulsion effect can be used positively as a mental conditioning exercise to develop the resilience to reject foods that are not conducive to living a healthy and long life.

Here is an example. Imagine a dead rat lying at the side of the road. Its belly has been split open and its guts have spilled out. Hundreds of maggots are feeding on the juicy find. Then notice that the shape of the rat reminds you of the shape of a burger. Perhaps a burger is in fact a cross-section of the dead rat? My guess is that the clearer you visualise this image, the less you will want to bite into a hamburger the next time you have the option.

This powerful technique can be used to combat the mind games played by TV advertisers. Eating greasy, salty, sugary, chemical-laden food is not natural or healthy. To get around this, advertisers present images of enjoyment, sex appeal and fun to elicit a positive emotional response from the viewer, fooling your brain into associating that pleasant emotion with eating these products. For example, advertisers frequently use famous comedians to provide voiceovers because the listener is likely to already associate laughter and therefore pleasure with the voice that they hear, which in turn gets associated with the product. This all happens at a subconscious level of which we are usually completely unaware. Despite the fact that we consciously know that these foods will cause us harm and make us more vulnerable to a myriad of illnesses, we still associate sugary, salty and greasy foods with pleasure and fool ourselves into thinking that we want them.

This subconscious effect or habit persists because the closer we are to experiencing pleasure, the more likely we are to become obsessed with it. We focus exclusively on the pleasure and decide that we want it again. We remember all the enjoyment and forget about all the negative effects. As we replay the pleasure experience in our minds, the sense of anticipation increases. It is like a drug addict focusing on the pleasure of feeding their craving while ignoring the detrimental effect on their health, the loss of money, the pain of withdrawal and the harmful effects on friends and family. If they could look at the complete picture they would probably never contemplate using drugs. Similarly, with harmful foods if we saw the entire picture we would never want to consume them again.

People usually try to combat compulsive eating in the moments before eating the food; however, this is the hardest time to try to combat the compulsion. It is easier to prepare yourself to defeat the compulsion when you are out walking or watching TV.

The Power of Revulsion

The useful thing about the revulsion effect is that it can be created and amplified at will, to the point of nausea and prepared for later use. The earlier example was of the similarities between a dead rat and a burger. Think of that burger again. It probably still carries the feelings of nausea that you associated with the thoughts of eating the dead rat.

You can use the revulsion effect to help you stop eating the harmful foods that you may have so far eaten habitually. The technique enables you to exit the obsession cycle and gives you the chance to focus on your good health and longevity goals.

Whenever you encounter a food that you want to give up, simply cultivate the feeling of revulsion by focusing on something that makes you feel nauseous. Leave the food aside and get moving. There is no harsh battle of will, no fighting obsession, just one moment of nausea and then off you go. Each time you conquer a harmful food craving you will be stronger for the next time you encounter that food.

Creating the revulsion effect is simple. With just a little practice, you will be able to create the feeling quickly and easily. Practise using it. Open the refrigerator door, create revulsion, then do something else. Use it several times a day, for two or three days, and it will soon become a hugely powerful tool that will put you in complete control of your food choices.

When to Use Revulsion

- When you are not hungry but are thinking about food.
- When you are overeating.
- While visualising the foods you are trying to quit eating.

Some Sample Revulsion Thoughts to Conquer Food Addictions

- French fries: Visualise old, parasite-ridden potatoes being sliced and dipped in two-week-old fat.
- Margarine: Imagine a factory worker filling the plastic tub while snot drips down into the container, mixing with the margarine.
- Red meat: Visualise a terrified animal being slaughtered and see yourself gorging on the animal flesh while it is still warm, in the midst of other screaming animals.
- Soft drinks: Teeth-dissolving and stomach-rotting liquid.
- Milk: Visualise suckling on a cow's udder.

The Live-Long Code Environmental Detox

We are exposed to harmful levels of chemicals and pollutants every day. When you imagine harmful pollutants you might visualise industrial chimney smoke or a smoggy, polluted urban area. The truth, though, is that the most harmful toxic pollutants are found in our homes. Because of our regular proximity to them they go unnoticed, even though they potentially do more harm than that smoke-belching factory.

As well as the toxins we encounter in our food, we also come into contact with them through body creams, tanning lotions and many other beauty products, which contain a variety of chemicals that potentially compromise our immune systems and are therefore detrimental to longevity. You can't avoid all harmful chemicals, but it is possible to dramatically decrease your exposure by paying attention to the products that you use in your home and on your body. This exercise will again involve a clearout and will involve making quite big changes, but once done the benefits will be significant.

Make the following key changes:

- Remove tobacco smoke from your home. If any of your friends or family want to smoke, tell them they are free to do so outside. As second-hand tobacco smoke contains over 4,000 chemicals, many of which are carcinogenic, there is no place for it in your home. If you are the one producing these chemicals by smoking, follow the Live-Long Code Smoking Detox approach detailed in the next section.
- Clear out all your domestic cleaning products, as they generally contain a large quantity of toxic chemicals. Consider healthier alternatives such as vinegar and water for cleaning windows, lemon juice for cleaning dishes and bathroom areas and baking soda and water for cleaning ovens. Undiluted white vinegar can be used as a household disinfectant. There are now a number of environmentally safe cleaning products readily available. The Ecover brand has a variety of products that safely provide for all your domestic cleaning needs.

171

- Throw out all artificial air fresheners. Although they may smell pleasant, they emit toxic odours that can cause cancer; they contain such lethal substances as ethanol, formaldehyde, phenol and xylene. As an alternative use proper ventilation together with natural essential oils on flower-based potpourri.
- When using scented candles, make sure that they are made from plant or beeswax and that they contain only pure essential oils and not synthetic fragrances.
- Remember to use your kitchen exhaust fan and make sure that it is vented outside.
- Avoid exposure to all products that contain methylene chloride and benzene. Methylene chloride is found in paint strippers and aerosol paint spray and has been found to cause cancer in animals. Benzene, found in paint, has also been found to cause cancer in humans.
- If you are redecorating your living room, try to use natural furnishings that have not been treated with chemicals. Consider natural wood flooring as an alternative to carpets, which usually contain volatile organic compounds. If you already have a carpet and wish to have it cleaned, have it steam cleaned without the use of toxic chemicals.

The Live-Long Code Smoking Detox

If you want to increase your chances of living a long and healthy life, regaining your freedom from your smoking habit is perhaps one of the most important things that you can do. Smoking causes so much direct and indirect damage to your body that eliminating it must be given immediate priority. It makes no sense to start eating pure and healthy food while continuing to inhale literally thousands of toxic chemicals into your lungs.

When you stop smoking you immediately start to receive a 'health rebate'. You may be surprised at just how quickly you start to gain the benefits of stopping.

What Happens to Your Body When You Stop Smoking

Within 20 minutes after you smoke that last cigarette, your body begins a series of changes that continue for years.

- 20 minutes after quitting
  Your heart rate and blood pressure drop to levels close to what they were before your last cigarette. The temperature of your hands and feet increases, returning to normal.

- 12 hours after quitting
  Carbon monoxide level in your blood drops to normal.
  Oxygen level in your blood increases to normal.

- 24 hours after quitting
  Your heart attack risk begins to drop.

- 48 hours after quitting
  Nerve endings start to regrow.
  Ability to smell and taste is enhanced.

- 2 weeks to 3 months after quitting
  Your lung function improves by up to 30 per cent.
  Circulation improves.
  Walking becomes easier.

- 1 to 9 months after quitting
  Cilia regrow in lungs, increasing ability to handle mucus; cleans the lungs, lowering your risk of lung infections. Lungs start to function better.
  Your body's overall energy increases.

- 1 year after quitting
  Your added risk of coronary heart disease is half that of a smoker's.

- 5 years after quitting
  Your stroke risk is reduced to that of a non-smoker's.

How to Quit Smoking

The Live-Long Code offers powerful techniques that can help you remove nicotine from your life for good so that you can live longer and healthier. Use all the techniques regularly and you will soon see the health rewards that come from being a non-smoker.

In preparation for quitting, do the following:

- The first few days, drink *lots* of water and green tea to help flush out the nicotine and other poisons from your body.
- Announce to your friends and family that you are quitting and ask for their support and encouragement. You'll be surprised how much it can help to ask for support and how much motivation this will give you to succeed.
- Ask friends and family members not to smoke in your presence. Don't be afraid to ask. This is more important than you may realise.
- On your quit day, hide all ashtrays and destroy all your cigarettes. You have to decide you are quitting. It is amazing how many people come to me seeking help with giving up smoking and yet stare incredulously at me when I tell them to throw out their cigarettes.
- If there are any places in particular where you used to smoke, rearrange the layout of those places. Move the seats or change the location of the phone. Our brains create a lot of associations around smoking, but you can break them simply by making small changes.

Technique One

Good breathing technique has already been discussed. Deep breathing is perhaps the most powerful technique for anyone giving up smoking. If you feel any cravings for a cigarette, do the following three times.

- Inhale the deepest breath you can into your lungs and then, very slowly, exhale. Purse your lips so that the air comes out slowly.

• As you exhale, close your eyes, and let your chin slowly drop to your chest. Visualise all the tension leaving your body, slowly draining out of your fingers and toes, just flowing on out.

When you master this, you'll be able to use it for any stressful situation in which you find yourself in the future. It will be your greatest weapon for fighting cravings. The best thing is that each and every time you succeed with the technique, its power increases. It works because deep breathing reduces stress. Ironically, smokers often only breathe deeply when they are smoking. They mistakenly believe that the feeling of relaxation comes from the cigarette – in reality it comes from the deep breathing that accompanies it.

Technique Two

Get a sheet of paper and, choosing from the following list, write down the six main reasons you don't like smoking, why it's bad and why you want to stop.

1. Cigarette smoking makes smokers age prematurely. A smoker in her forties may have as many wrinkles as a non-smoker in her sixties.
2. Smoking increases the risk of impotence by around 5 per cent for men in their thirties and forties.
3. Female smokers have more trouble getting pregnant than non-smokers and also have a higher rate of miscarriages.
4. Smoking makes your breath, hair and clothes stink.
5. Teeth and fingers get stained brown with nicotine.
6. A typical pack-a-day smoker spends over £112/€130 a month and nearly £1,500/€1,700 a year.
7. One in five people dies from illnesses directly linked to smoking.
8. If you smoke regularly for a long time you may get a disease called peripheral vascular disease; this causes narrowing of the blood vessels, which restricts blood flow to the hands and feet, leading to gangrene and potentially to amputation.

9. Smoking messes up your body chemistry; for example, it decreases the vitamin C levels in your blood. Vitamin C protects against carcinogens, boosts immunity and helps prevent heart disease. Also, smoking increases cholesterol. It's estimated that every cigarette you smoke raises the level of bad cholesterol in your body.

10. Smokers have a higher frequency of severe depression, anxiety disorders and other psychological problems than non-smokers.

11. If you smoke you have an increased risk of gum disease, muscle injuries, angina, neck pain, back pain, abnormal eye movements, circulatory disease, fungal eye infection, ulcers, osteoporosis, cataracts, Crohn's disease, pneumonia, depression, psoriasis, type 2 diabetes, skin wrinkling, hearing loss, flu, rheumatoid arthritis, tendon injuries and ligament injuries – amongst other conditions.

12. Smoking causes cancer. The links between cigarettes and cancers of the oral cavity, oesophagus, lungs, kidneys, pancreas, stomach, cervix and bladder are indisputable.

Next, on the other side of the sheet, write down all the reasons why you'll feel great when you've succeeded in stopping smoking. For example, you'll feel healthier, your sense of taste and smell will be enhanced, your hair and clothes will smell fresher, and so on. When you have finished fold this sheet of paper and carry it where you used to carry your cigarettes.

Technique Three

Now let's apply the revulsion technique discussed earlier to re-programme your mind to feel a sense of disgust towards cigarettes. Recall four times when you have thought to yourself 'I've got to quit smoking', or when you felt disgusted about smoking. Maybe somebody you know was badly affected by smoking. Take a moment now to come up with four separate occasions when you felt that you had to quit or were disgusted by smoking.

Next close your eyes and remember each of those times as though they were happening right now. Jump from each memory to the next and keep going until you can make them all as vivid as possible. See what you saw, hear what you heard and feel how you felt. Take some time now and go through those memories again and again. Rapidly overlap each memory with the next until you feel totally and utterly disgusted by cigarettes.

Technique Four

Do you know, or know of, an adult who continues to carry around a blanket – or 'blankie' – that they had as a baby? The human mind is very sensitive to associations and in this case the person associated comfort and safety with the blanket as an infant. Subconsciously they have fooled themselves into continuing to believe that this sense of comfort emanates from the blanket itself.

In a similar way people become accustomed to having cigarettes in certain situations. For example, if you smoke while taking a break and chatting to work colleagues, subconsciously you fool yourself into thinking that the relaxation of taking a break and the enjoyment of talking to friends is due to the cigarette. This of course is just as irrational as the notion of someone's 'blankie' being a source of safety. So now that you have quit smoking, continue to award yourself relaxation time – but do something different. Go for a walk or chat with a friend.

Technique Five

Several times a day, quietly repeat to yourself the affirmation 'I am a non-smoker.' Many quitters see themselves as smokers who are just not smoking for the moment. Silently repeating the affirmation 'I am a non-smoker' will help you change your view of yourself, and even if it may seem silly to you, this is actually a very useful and very powerful technique. Use it!

Technique Six

You used to use cigarettes as a signal to your body to release happy chemicals, so next let's programme some powerfully positive feelings into your future. Sit comfortably and recall a time when you felt very deep pleasure. Take a moment to remember it as vividly as possible. Remember the detail – see what you saw, hear what you heard and feel how good you felt.

Keep going through the memory, then as soon as it finishes, go through it again and again, all the time squeezing your thumb and forefinger together. Make the pictures big, bright and vivid, the sounds loud and crisp and the feelings strong. Again squeeze your thumb and forefinger together. This creates an associational link between the squeeze of your fingers and that great feeling.

OK, now stop and relax. If you have done the exercise correctly, whenever you squeeze your thumb and finger together you should feel that good feeling again. Try that now – squeeze thumb and finger and remember that good feeling. Keep practising it over and over.

Now you are going to programme good feelings to happen automatically whenever you are in a situation where you used to smoke.

Squeeze your thumb and finger together, get that great feeling going and now imagine being in a situation where you would have smoked, *but* instead you are there, feeling great, without a cigarette. See what you'll see, hear what you'll hear, and take that good feeling into those situations without the need for a cigarette.

Imagine a situation where you are offered a cigarette and smile broadly and confidently, saying, 'No thanks, I don't smoke.' And notice how you feel good about it!

A significant point that you should bear in mind is that a few weeks after quitting, any urge to smoke will subside considerably. At this stage it's important to understand that occasionally, you may still get a desire for 'just one cigarette'. This could happen out of the blue, perhaps during moments of stress, whether negative stress or positive (for example, at a party or on holiday). If you are un-prepared to resist, succumbing to that 'one cigarette' may lead you directly back to smoking. So be ready and be strong.

Summary

- By banishing unhealthy habits you will significantly improve your health and extend your life expectancy. Begin your detox by performing the Live-Long Code Kitchen Clearout to set yourself on the way to vibrant good health. The revulsion technique on page 167 will help you to implement the Live-Long Code Nutrition Plan.
- Try to use healthier cooking methods like steaming and stir-frying and avoid cooking materials that can expose you to toxic residues.
- Focus on your oral health. Having clean and healthy teeth and gums not only makes you look better, but also protects you against heart disease. Consider having any mercury removed from your mouth by a dental specialist, and certainly avoid all future amalgam fillings.
- Stop smoking and avoid exposure to second-hand smoke. Smoking is one of the biggest human killers, taking millions of lives by way of heart disease, lung disease and cancer, amongst other things. Use the techniques in this chapter to free yourself from this habit for good.

If you have already reduced your exposure to harmful chemical toxins, your body will be stronger and healthier from day one of the detox. You will have boosted your immunity and dramatically reduced your risk exposure to a variety of diseases and conditions. In the next chapter you will learn how by just taking 3.5 hours of exercise a week you will not only improve your health but also develop the body of an 'immortal'. Let's now look at the most powerful exercise system for turning back the clock.

CHAPTER SIX

The Live-Long Code Exercise Programme

What To Do And Why You Must Do It

When you ask people if they would like to live to be 100 or more, most don't give the answer you'd expect. For a lot of people the fear of disability and helplessness is greater than the fear of death, and truthfully this fear is quite reasonable. By the time most people reach 85, there's a 50 per cent likelihood of needing help to perform such simple daily tasks as bathing, walking, dressing, cooking, shopping, even going to the toilet. Most of us dread the notion of ending up in a nursing home. But it doesn't have to be like this. How do we prevent falling into helplessness when we reach old age? The answer is exercise.

To prepare for a long and healthy life, the first priority is to remain strong. The next priority is to retain balance and co-ordination. For older people, falls are a leading cause of disability and even death. Approximately one-third of people over the age of 65 take a fall each year. This figure rises as age increases, with over half of people aged over 80 falling at least once a year. For older people, weaker bones are more likely to break in a fall, and a staggering 20 per cent of those who suffer a hip fracture die within 12 months. For survivors, the chance of ending up in a nursing home increases by over 500 per cent.

Exercise plays a vital role in keeping you strong and steady on your feet as you gain years. By keeping muscles toned, improving posture and balance, and extending your range of motion, a proper exercise programme can help maintain strength and vitality for many years. There are many forms of exercise that support active ageing: tai chi and chi kung are probably the most well known and popular examples of an exercise system that dramatically improves balance and considerably reduces the chances of falling for those who practise it. Walking is also something that I call a miracle exercise; a recent study found that people who walked regularly reduced their risk of hip fracture by 30 per cent.

A 2005 Harvard study of 2,987 women noted that walking for just 25 to 45 minutes a day approximately doubled the survival rate in breast cancer patients. Numerous other studies have indicated that walking for half an hour every day can protect against a variety of cancers and heart disease by as much as 50 per cent.

Exercise is an amazing elixir of youth and a key element of the Live-Long Code. The Live-Long Code's suggested amount of exercise is 30 minutes every day of the week. Most people do not take enough exercise and approximately 25 per cent of people do not take any exercise at all. If you are currently one of these people, now is the time for you to change that.

In this chapter you will learn a revolutionary training approach that multiplies the beneficial effect of training such that these 30 minutes each day are more efficient and effective than spending many hours training each day. Your training schedule is as follows.

	Sun	Mon	Tue	Wed	Thur	Fri	Sat
Flexibility	5 mins	5 mins	5 mins	5 mins	5 mins	5 mins	5 mins
Strength		15 mins		15 mins		15 mins	
Cardiovascular		10 mins		10 mins		10 mins	
Walking	25 mins		25 mins		25 mins		25 mins

In the past, the majority of people's lives were full of physical activity. For the longest-living people in the world – the Okinawans of Japan, who we have looked at briefly already – this is still the case. For most Okinawans, transport consists of their own two feet. Many of their occupations still require a high degree of physical activity throughout the day.

The computer age and modern Western development have radically changed the way we live and the amount of physical activity that is part of the average person's day. Technology has started doing the hard jobs at work and at home, and our free time is now often spent in front of a television or a computer. We have become used to a sedentary lifestyle, where we move as little as possible throughout the day. This lifestyle starves your body of energy and vitality.

Leading health experts all recognise the importance of exercise and generally agree that as little as 30 minutes of the *right* exercise will make all the difference to both the way you feel now and the way you will feel when you are older. I emphasise the word *right*, because while the duration of training is relatively short, the focus and the intensity should be high. We are frequently reminded of how important it is to plan financially for our retirement. Think of your health in the same way; by exercising just a little every day, not only will you start to feel much better immediately, you will also be preparing for healthy and rewarding later years. Short exercise sessions are just as beneficial as long ones, as long as you get at least 30 to 40 minutes of exercise in total every day. This includes making small choices like talking a walk on your lunch break or using the stairs instead of the lift. Done frequently, these all add up to significant health gains.

Although the Live-Long Code Exercise Programme is vigorous, it is not exhausting. It incorporates the right mix and balance of exercise activities: flexibility training to support strength and balance, cardiovascular exercise to condition the heart and cardiovascular system and strength training to maintain strong muscles and bones.

Flexibility and Balance Work

As we have seen, the most common cause of disability in people aged 85 and older involves problems with balance. Falls for people in their eighties must therefore be ranked alongside heart disease, cancer and dementia as one of the top health concerns.

Stretching offers several significant benefits. As well as improving posture and releasing muscular tension, stretching can provide protection against injury. Supple muscles and elastic tendons are key elements to retaining dexterity. Stretching also strengthens and supports the lower back muscles, which helps to minimise back problems, an issue of increasing importance as we get older.

Stretching contributes to improving your balance overall, but there are also specific exercises you can do to improve your body's stability. The ancient exercise systems of chi kung and tai chi have great power to improve your health. These systems have been proven to improve balance, increase muscle strength, lower blood pressure and reduce stress. No matter what age you are, these are exercises that you can start – and continue – for a lifetime.

There are also several other systems that offer stretching and balance training. Pilates uses slow exercises that target the stomach and back muscles to strengthen your 'core'. Yoga, the Indian system of held postures, is growing in popularity and classes are now within easy reach for most people.

Strength Training for Muscle and Bone Mass

It is never too late to start strength training. Developing and reserving muscle mass is an important aspect of staying youthful as we grow older. For most people, muscle size and strength reaches its peak during the twenties and then starts a downward trend that for some people can lead to difficulty getting around or even getting up out of a chair. This decline, however, is not inevitable! Scientists have investigated what elements cause this downward spiral. Is this loss of muscle mass caused by an enzyme, a gene or another biological factor? The reality is much simpler than that. As we age, we generally use our muscles less and less. The principle is use it or lose it. The solution is a simple one – use it! And use it by doing strength training.

I can hear some protests already. 'I don't want to end up looking like Arnold Schwarzenegger!' That's not what we are talking about here. Just as there are several ways of achieving better aerobic fitness, you don't have to add masses of muscular bulk to increase your strength. Strength training, whether you do it by using equipment or by other means, offers very effective prevention of many diseases and disorders, along with a nice improvement in your physical appearance.

And as well as improving the way you feel physically, strength training will improve your mental state. A Harvard Medical School study has shown that a progressive resistance training programme can be an effective antidepressant. Working out with weights releases endorphins, the 'happy brain' hormones that improve your sense of well being.

Cardiovascular Exercise for a Healthy Heart

Cardiovascular activity, which raises the heart rate through vigorous movement, can keep your cardiovascular system young and healthy, helping to ward off heart attacks and other cardiovascular conditions – conditions that are the leading cause of mortality in the Western world.

Cardiovascular exercise also burns calories, which helps with weight management. It lowers your blood pressure, improves your metabolism, enhances your sleep and often dramatically improves your mood. Cardiovascular workouts can be as easy as walking with friends, salsa dancing with your partner or enjoying a social game of tennis.

- A 22–year study of 2,014 men in midlife found that physical fitness was a strong predictor of mortality. Even small improvements in exercise habits significantly lowered the risk of death for these men in their peak productivity years.
- One of the most exciting findings of the MacArthur Foundation Study of Successful Ageing has been that the senior participants who were physically active had the best-preserved mental function 10 years later. This is important evidence that a sound body and mind go hand in hand for life.

- Another aspect of the MacArthur study looked at how twins fared in relation to their aerobic exercise habits. Aerobics blew genetics away. Individuals who walked briskly or jogged for 30 minutes just six times a month had a 40 per cent lower risk of dying than their twins who did not exercise. So take heart if you come from a family with a history of cardiovascular disease or other killer illnesses. Regular cardiovascular exercise (and good health habits) can outweigh your genetic endowment.

Make no mistake about it, each of the components of exercise discussed here is equally important. It is well known that aerobics is good for the heart. What is less well known, but just as important, is that flexibility training and strength training contribute just as much to longevity. As you read on, you will come to a better understanding of the reasons why. Suffice it to say at this point that any anti-ageing exercise programme must be individually tailored to meet your personal needs, based on your current physical condition. The programme must also include a balance of the three components mentioned above.

Let's now look at each of the three components in detail.

The Live-Long Code Flexibility Training Programme

A loss of flexibility is a significant part of physical ageing and a critical consideration in the Live-Long Code Programme. Some people make the mistake of going straight into exercise without warming up the body and stretching their muscles. Not taking the time to stretch the muscles is missing out on an important element of any anti-ageing exercise programme. Even if you do understand the importance of stretching, though, you still need to know how to go about it effectively and safely. You must learn exactly how to incorporate stretching into your schedule while at the same time letting it take up no more than 10 minutes a day.

Flexibility training is the foundation of your exercise programme because it helps to increase blood supply to the muscles. It also warms up the key muscle groups and makes the body more supple and far less prone to injury. The message is simple: do not start any weight training or aerobic programme without stretching properly first.

The flexibility training programme is straightforward to follow and, once you get used to it, it will become second nature. It is recommended that you follow the sequence as laid out in the programme.

Stretch One: Chest

Posture
- Grip a pole or doorway with your left hand thumb up at chest level.
- Stand with feet shoulder width apart.
- Keep your knees slightly bent.

Performance
- Exhale slowly as you turn your torso towards the left.
- Hold your stretch for 3 seconds.
- Ease out of the stretch and inhale.
- Perform for 5 repetitions and then change to the right side.

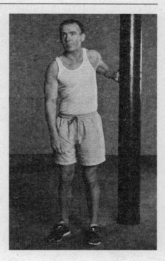

Stretch Two: Back

Posture
- Place both feet at the bottom of a sturdy pole.
- Grip the pole with both hands at waist level.

Performance
- Exhale slowly as you allow your hips to move backwards. Feel your back stretching.
- Maintain a slight bend in your elbows and knees.
- Hold your stretch for 3 seconds before returning to the standing position.
- Perform 5 repetitions.

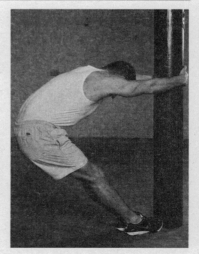

Stretch Three: Shoulders

Posture
- Stand with feet shoulder width apart.
- Bring your right arm across your chest while keeping your neck and shoulder muscles relaxed.
- Place your left hand just behind the right elbow.

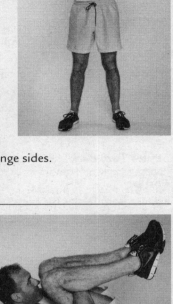

Performance
- As you exhale, slowly pull on your right am with your left hand.
- Hold the stretch for 3 seconds.
- Release your right arm as you inhale.
- Perform 5 repetitions and then change sides.

Stretch Four: Lower Back

Posture
- Lie down in a face-up position.
- Hug your knees to your chest and bring your chin to your knees.

Performance
- As you exhale, pull your legs and chest towards each other.
- Hold the stretch for 3 seconds.
- While inhaling ease out of the stretch, allowing your feet and back to return to the floor.
- Perform 5 repetitions.

Stretch Five: Mid, Lower and Upper Back

Posture
- Get down on your hands and knees so you resemble a cat.
- Place your wrists under your shoulders and knees under your hips with your back straight.

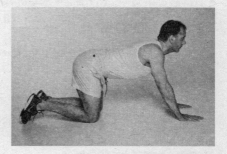

Performance
- Allow your abdomen to slowly drop down, allowing your lower back to bend downward, and stretch. Hold this position for 15 seconds.
- Next, slowly arch your back as much as possible and hold for at least 5 seconds.

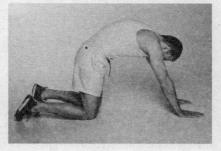

- Sit back on your heels with arms extended out straight. Hold again for 5–10 seconds.
- A well-performed cat stretch takes a little time to master. Take your time to perfect it.

Stretch Six: Spine, Hips and Lower Back

Posture
- Lie down on your back, keeping your feet on the floor and knees bent.
- Bring your arms out to the sides.

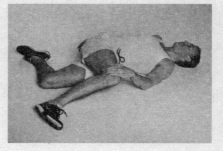

189

Performance

- Lower your knees to the left as you exhale.
- Extend your right leg beyond your left leg, allowing the stretch to extend.
- Place your left hand on your right knee and press gently.
- Hold the stretch for 3 seconds.
- Ease out the stretch while inhaling and bringing your knees back to the centre.
- Perform 5 repetitions and then change sides and repeat.

Stretch Seven: Quadriceps

Posture

- Stand approximately 2 feet away from a wall.
- Position your left hand against the wall for balance.

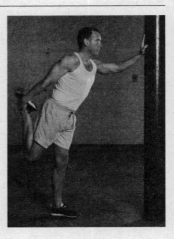

Performance

- As you exhale, raise your right foot backwards towards your buttocks.
- Hold your right foot with your right hand.
- Lean forward as you pull your leg backwards, pressing your heel towards your buttocks.
- Keep your right knee slightly bent.
- Pull gently until you feel a strong stretch and then hold for 3 seconds.
- While inhaling, release your left leg and allow it to return to the floor.
- Perform 5 repetitions and then switch sides.

Stretch Eight: Hamstring

Posture

- Lie on your back, face up.
- Bend your right knee and keep your left leg resting on the floor.

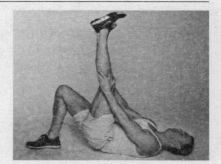

Performance

- As you exhale, raise your left leg upwards.
- Keep your leg straight and hold it at the knee.
- Pull gently until you feel it stretch behind your knee and along your thigh.
- Hold the stretch for 10 seconds.
- Repeat on the other side.

Stretch Nine: Biceps

Posture

- Stand upright with your feet shoulder width apart.
- Grasp a pole or the side of a door at chest level with your left hand, thumb down.

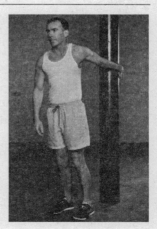

Performance

- As you exhale, slowly turn away from the bar until you feel a comfortable stretch in your biceps.
- Hold for 3 seconds.
- While inhaling, ease out the stretch.
- Perform for 5 repetitions and then switch sides.

Stretch Ten: Triceps

Posture

- Stand with feet shoulder width apart.
- Bring your right arm overhead, with your elbow bent and hand behind the neck.
- Place your left hand on the right elbow.

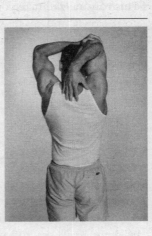

Performance

- As you exhale, slowly pull your right elbow with your left hand.
- Hold the stretch for 3 seconds.
- While inhaling, release your right arm.
- Perform 5 repetitions and then switch sides.

Stretch Eleven: Calves

Posture

- Stand in front of a stationary object like a wall.
- Place your left foot in front and your right foot behind you.
- Place the toes of the right foot on a slightly elevated object – 2 inches high.

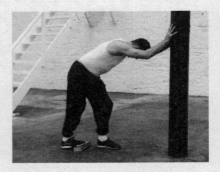

Performance

- As you exhale, lean forward, moving your weight onto your left leg.
- Press your right heel down onto the floor as you do this.
- Straighten out your right leg and stretch for 3 seconds.
- While inhaling, relax your right leg.
- Perform 5 repetitions before changing sides.

This routine will take you approximately 5 minutes. Make sure to do it slowly and to allow a full range of movement during each stretch. Shake the muscle you have stretched loose after each exercise. Ensure that your muscles feel loose and relaxed before you move on to any aerobic or weight training exercises. It is also recommended that during the strength training programme, you perform the stretches associated with the muscle group you're working in each exercise before and after you perform the weight lifting, as part of your warm-up and cool-down. Push yourself to the limit of each stretch and your flexibility will increase.

How Often Should You Stretch?

Stretching should be done on a daily basis. It is easy to do and can be done anywhere and without any special equipment. It can be done at any time of the day to relieve any muscular tension, but it is especially recommended in the morning, or before exercising.

Flexibility Training and Ageing

You will benefit from flexibility training no matter how old you are. In fact, the older you are, the more attention you should pay to flexibility training; perhaps perform it more than once a day. Flexibility declines after the age of about 25 due to a decrease in the size of the muscle fibres and the connective ligaments and tendons associated with them. An individual's level of activity will also affect their flexibility. People who are more active generally have greater flexibility than those who are not. Inactivity causes shortening and contraction of muscle fibres, which in turn leads to inflexibility. Regular stretching therefore increases the functionality of your skeletal system and increases healthy longevity.

The Importance of Combining Flexibility Training with Cardiovascular and Strength Training

It is probably obvious by now that flexibility training must be performed as an integral part of any anti-ageing programme.

Flexibility training is therefore a cornerstone of the Live-Long Code Exercise Programme. This section has hopefully enabled you to understand the logic of flexibility training, but knowledge must be put into action. Take action now and commence your Live-Long Code Flexibility Programme – and maintain it as part of your daily exercise routine.

Strength Training

Anti-ageing experts generally agree that strength training must be an integral part of any exercise programme. There is a good reason for this: as we age our muscular body mass decreases by up to 10 per cent with each decade after the age of 30. This means that by the age of 70 most people will have only retained 50 per cent of their muscle strength. This decrease in body strength ultimately leads to a decrease in muscular function, a loss of energy, impaired balance and a consequent increase in accident rate. Increasing strength therefore has to be a cornerstone of the Live-Long Code Exercise Programme.

Strength Training for Any Age

A Tufts University of Boston study from 1994 showed the remarkable benefits of strength training. Dr Maria Fiatarone gave nutritional supplements and an exercise training programme to a group of people aged between 63 and 98 who were living in a nursing home. Eighty-three per cent of these people required a cane, walker or a wheelchair and 66 per cent of them had a history of falls.

Every participant in the study went through a high-intensity, progressive strength training programme for 45 minutes, three times a week. After just 10 weeks, the results were nothing less than astounding. The muscular strength of the subjects had increased by an amazing 174 per cent on average, with the most notable benefits coming to those who had been weakest to begin with. There was also a significant improvement in mobility, with most subjects able to walk faster and climb steps much more comfortably. The average walking speed of the group increased by over 50 per cent and after taking part in the programme some of the individuals no longer needed the assistance of a walker. It is astonishing that something so simple and non-medical could have such a staggering effect; surely if any pharmaceutical had achieved these results it would be hailed as a wonder drug!

Exercise and Natural Growth Hormone Production

When we perform strength training exercises, it sends a signal to the pituitary gland to release growth hormone – which is key to anti-ageing. While we don't fully understand why this happens, it is beyond any doubt that it does happen and that it has significant benefits for increasing lifespan. Cardiovascular exercise yields a similar release of growth hormone.

During strength training at 70 per cent of maximum lift, a similar amount of growth hormone is released as during cardiovascular training at 70 per cent of maximum heart rate. If the weight lifted is increased to 85 per cent of maximum capacity, the amount of growth hormone released increases by an enormous 400 per cent.

The Benefits of Strength Training

Strength training is for many people associated with bodybuilding and an Arnold Schwarzenegger physique. That is not our goal with strength training – and it will not happen to you unless you are foolish enough to start using anabolic steroids. Some women are concerned that by doing strength training they will develop a masculine physique. The women who develop such masculine physiques exercise to the extreme and most of them use performance enhancing drugs. This will not happen here. The result of the Live-Long Code Strength Training Programme will be an increase in physical performance and a measurable improvement in your strength. Stronger muscles enable you to move better and improve your endurance. This is especially beneficial to post-menopausal women, who have an increased risk of osteoporosis. Our muscles serve as a supporting structure for our skeletal framework, so strong muscles improve balance and mean fewer accidents. From an anti-ageing perspective, our aim is to replace fat with muscle, leaving you with greater muscle tone and lean mass.

It is normal during a strength training programme to gain a few pounds of muscle as well as increase your strength by up to 50 per cent after just 12 weeks of consistent training. A strength training programme will change your body composition, and this change will have a direct effect on your appearance, giving you a much firmer and more toned look.

How Weight Training Stimulates Metabolism

We know that, as we get older, we generally lose about half a pound of muscle every year. This in turn lowers our metabolic rate, which means we need fewer calories to maintain our body's functions. This means that if we consume the same amount of food as earlier in our lives, the surplus calories will be stored as fat. This is why most people notice that they are getting fatter and less muscular as they get older. Unless you exercise and adjust your diet this will be the natural and inevitable course of events. If you want to retain or indeed develop a more youthful body composition, you have to include a strength training programme in your exercise schedule.

Strength Training Terminology

Exercise – describes the complete strength training movement for the muscle group being strengthened. For example, the biceps curl is an exercise.

Repetitions, or reps – one full movement of the exercise, from start to the prescribed endpoint and back to the original starting position, is called a rep.

Set – refers to a complete number of reps. For example, doing a bench press 12 consecutive times will complete one set. There are usually one to three sets in one exercise routine. The pause between sets is usually 1 to 1½ minutes, which enables the exercised muscles to recover so they can complete the next set effectively.

Positive phase – the phase of the exercise that requires your muscles to contract. When you are doing a bench press, for example, the positive phase is when you press the weight upwards, away from your body.

Negative phase – the phase when you are slowly allowing the weight to return to home position. For example, for the biceps curl, the negative phase is when you slowly lower the weight back down until your arms extend straight.

Strength Training Frequency and Duration

Cutting-edge studies show that you can perform strength training exercises very briefly – perhaps for just 15 minutes three times a week – and this is sufficient to develop significant strength and muscle. Strength training does not have to be complicated; all good gyms today have machines that simplify weight training. You can choose from a variety of forms of strength training, depending on the type of equipment you have at your disposal. I do recommend that you join a gym to get the advantage of guidance from the professionals there, as the scope of this book does not extend to detailing all the strength training possibilities or how to tailor your programme as your strength and condition improve.

Strength Training in a Gym

Gyms usually have many machines that make it easier to train with weights. Gym machinery enables you to do exercises that involve isolating specific muscles and therefore exercising them with greater focus and intensity. Having a gym membership is an excellent investment for your health and longevity. As well as machines, though, barbells and dumbbells (known as free weights) also work your muscles in different and beneficial ways. Free weights are still considered by many to be the best way to achieve results. By combining free weights and machines you can create a very effective strength training programme.

When Your Muscles Are Sore

If you have not exercised for a while it is normal to feel soreness and aching in your muscles after training. This pain is due to the muscle breaking down and is a normal healthy process; the muscle will rebuild itself stronger. However, the pain is also a signal to your body that you need to rest the muscle. It is only during this rest period that the muscle grows and develops. It is important, therefore, to give yourself at least a day's rest between weight training, during which the pain will usually subside. If the pain does not go away you may need to rest some more between sessions, at least initially. If the pain still does not go away after a few days, it is sensible to consult your doctor for further evaluation.

Any sudden-onset pain during exercise is not normal. If there is a popping sound or a very severe pain you should stop immediately and get medical advice. By training slowly and with the guidance of a fitness coach, however, you are likely to avoid this. Muscular cramps are due to overexertion and can be caused by inadequate stretching or warming up of the muscle. It is also important to keep hydrated before and during exercise, as dehydration can contribute to cramps.

Improper training can result in injury or damage to your tendons and ligaments. This is why I recommend that you get the guidance of a fitness instructor when performing this or any strength training programme. If you do get injured, prolonged rest and medical attention are required. It is counterproductive from any perspective, including an anti-ageing one, to sustain injuries in training, so you should take every step to avoid injury.

Stretching Before Strength Training

To prevent injury and improve performance, you must warm up before your strength training exercise. At first, make sure that you use weights that you can handle. It is also important to cool down after strength training so that you avoid lightheadedness. A gradual cooling down helps to safely return your body to a relaxed state.

Strength Training Techniques

Strength-training programmes involve pressuring the muscles in a structured and organised way. Your programme should be easy for you to understand and follow. Here are some of the main points you should remember when developing your programme:

1. Start by exercising the larger muscle groups such as the chest, upper back, legs, biceps and triceps.
2. Do not overeat before or after performing your exercises. Eating too much before exercising reduces the blood supply to the muscles, as the blood is diverted to the stomach and intestines to aid digestion. Eating too soon after exercising has a similar effect.
3. However, it is important to have enough energy for strength training; try not to work out on an empty stomach either.
4. A good strength training programme requires an even powering of muscles throughout the exercise. This is easier to achieve if you perform each exercise slowly. A frequent mistake made by people beginning strength training is to use weights that are too heavy, lift them too fast and use a jerking motion. Each exercise has a positive phase where the muscle is contracted and a negative phase where the muscle is returned to its original state.

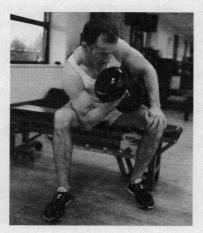

Knowing What Weight to Use

Everybody's muscles are different and the size and strength of your muscles are related not to the amount of work done, but rather to the amount of work done in a short unit of time i.e., or intensity. As an example, a marathon runner uses their muscles more than a sprinter because they run for much longer periods. However, when you compare intensity, the sprinter runs 30 feet per second compared to the marathon runner, who runs 18 feet per second. The difference is the intensity of use; sprinters develop larger muscles than marathon runners.

The most effective and efficient way to increase muscle strength is by performing strength training exercise with maximum strength and high intensity. In the 1950s the German physiologist Erich A. Muller discovered that performing just one set and one repetition of an exercise for no more than 6 seconds, with the weight held at maximum muscular contraction, was far more effective than performing multiple repetitions and multiple sets. The key is that you lift as heavy a weight as possible for this short duration, maximising the intensity of the exercise. With this method of training the average increase in muscle strength is 5 per cent a week.

It doesn't matter how much a muscle is used, it will not get stronger or larger unless it is overloaded. This means that you have to work the muscle intensively, and as its strength increases you have to increase the resistance in order for the improvement to continue.

When you begin your strength training programme, you will probably have no idea what weight to use for each exercise, so I would suggest that you use your first couple of sessions to determine how much weight you can handle. Simply lift the weight until your muscle is fully contracted. If you can lift the weight into position easily it is probably too light. Keep adding a small amount of weight until you need to use your maximum effort to lift the weight into position and hold it for 6 seconds. Once you are able to hold the weight at maximum contraction for more than 10 seconds you should increase the weight by between 5 and 10 per cent in your next session. To do this properly you need to keep a proper training log and accurately record what weight you lift in each exercise, in every session. You might well be surprised by how fast your strength increases; lifting 30 kg might prove very difficult in the first week, but you may find as soon as your second week that you can lift 40 kg relatively easily.

It is advisable to perform your exercises slowly and deliberately, with no sudden jerky movements. If you have someone to train with, they can help you to lift your weights to your fully contracted position.

Having a clear understanding of the basic principles of proper exercise performance, together with an understanding of how muscles contract, can make the difference between simply wasting many gym hours and fulfilling your goals in a very short time. For anti-ageing purposes, the main goal is to increase strength and stimulate growth hormone secretion; training with relatively heavy weights and decreasing the repetitions is the optimum approach for anti-ageing purposes.

How Often Should You Strength Train?

The Live-Long Code recommends three strength training workouts per week, approximately 15 minutes per session, each immediately followed by a short intensive cardiovascular session. On each day in between strength training sessions, I recommend that you walk briskly for 25 minutes.

How to Breathe When Strength Training

Inhale during the start of the lift, pause your breath and then exhale as you finish the lift. For example, when you are doing a bench press, inhale as you lower the weight to your chest. Pause your breath as you begin to press the weight up. Finish the exercise by exhaling during the latter part of the movement. The same goes for other strength training exercises.

Special Considerations for Women

1. **Menstruation**

   Overtraining can lead to a condition known as amenorrhea in which menstruation stops. If this happens it is a sign that you are overtraining and you should cut back. Once you do this the condition generally cures itself.

2. **Pregnancy**

   It's important to keep fit during pregnancy as this will usually facilitate a more comfortable and healthy pregnancy and sometimes a shorter labour. However, very strenuous activity during pregnancy should be avoided. The level of training should reduce as the pregnancy advances. You can increase training again gradually after the birth.

Measuring Your Progress

It is best to measure your progress by how well you feel. Anti-ageing exercises should lead to greater muscle tone, a reduced loss of muscle mass and a reduction in body fat. Depending on your size to begin with, you may in fact put weight on. Pure weight loss is therefore not a barometer of success; if you are achieving the other results then you are on target with your goals.

The Importance of Combining Stretching, Cardio-Vascular and Strength Training Exercises

By now it is probably very clear that strength training is an integral part of the Live-Long Code Exercise Programme. Strength training combats ageing and increases your life expectancy. Strength training should, however, be carried out alongside cardiovascular exercises as well as the stretching exercises covered earlier.

Staying Motivated

Initially you should be motivated because you will be excited by the challenge of the exercise programme. The real benefits, however, come from staying with the programme. Using metrics to gauge your progress is one method to help yourself stay motivated. Check cholesterol, body fat and blood pressure levels and monitor them every few weeks to confirm that you are making progress. Setting goals is an important aspect of many parts of our lives, exercise being no exception. Set goals that are measurable and achievable. Anti-ageing is a lifelong process with lifelong benefits.

Your First Strength Training Workout

The most important goal of any workout is to avoid injury. If you are new to the gym, you will need time to get to know the equipment and the techniques for each exercise. Ask for guidance from the staff. Feel free to use lighter weights to begin with until you fully understand how the physical movement machines and equipment work.

Here are some guidelines:

- Take your time to familiarise yourself with each exercise. Use bars or machines with no weight at all until you familiarise yourself with the technique of the exercise.
- Focus on the targeted muscle during each exercise so that you can really feel that muscle working.
- Maintain good posture while performing all exercises. This will help prevent injury to your back.
- Train within your capabilities for the first few workouts until the exercise action is firmly fixed in your mind.

When you finish your first session, congratulate yourself on a job well done and look forward to continuing on the road to increased health and longevity.

Guidelines for the First Month's Training

The most important part of the first month of training is to establish good exercise form and focus on understanding the exercises, trying to create good habits from the outset. You may or may not see significant improvements in this first month; the real key is to keep up the momentum for the months ahead and into the future. Follow these recommendations:

- Train three times a week with weights, and three times a week with cardio, for no more than 30 minutes each session.
- When strength training, work only to your plan; don't get over-enthusiastic and start switching around.
- Get guidance from your gym's fitness instructor. They are paid and trained to help you.
- Listen to your body. Certain days will feel better than others for your body. If you are feeling particularly tired, still try to train, but reduce the duration and intensity.
- Make sure you are also following the rest of the Live-Long Code and eating well, sleeping well and taking the right supplements.

The following programme works on all of the major muscle groups. When you have mastered the techniques, work on performing the exercises in quick succession with only short rest periods. This is a simple but fantastic workout to begin with as it creates a power-ful metabolic response, which stimulates muscle growth. Because you perform only short rests between exercises you produce a lot of blood lactate, which increases the production of human growth hormone – which is the key to exercising for anti-ageing.

It's also a good idea to change your training routine at least every four to six weeks. To alter your workout after the first six weeks you can seek assistance from a qualified personal trainer or refer to the Live-Long Code website www.immortalitycode.com for ongoing guidance and assistance.

Immortality Code Training Log

Date	dd/mm/yy										
Leg extension	kg	kg	kg	kg	kg	kg	kg	kg	kg	kg	kg
Leg curls	kg	kg	kg	kg	kg	kg	kg	kg	kg	kg	kg
Calf raises	kg	kg	kg	kg	kg	kg	kg	kg	kg	kg	kg
Lateral pulldowns	kg	kg	kg	kg	kg	kg	kg	kg	kg	kg	kg
Shrugs	kg	kg	kg	kg	kg	kg	kg	kg	kg	kg	kg
Cable crossovers	kg	kg	kg	kg	kg	kg	kg	kg	kg	kg	kg
Lateral raises	kg	kg	kg	kg	kg	kg	kg	kg	kg	kg	kg
Bent over laterals	kg	kg	kg	kg	kg	kg	kg	kg	kg	kg	kg
Tricep kickbacks	kg	kg	kg	kg	kg	kg	kg	kg	kg	kg	kg
Crunches	kg	kg	kg	kg	kg	kg	kg	kg	kg	kg	kg
Close grip chin	kg	kg	kg	kg	kg	kg	kg	kg	kg	kg	kg

The Live-Long Code

Exercise One — Leg Extension

Sit on the leg extension machine so that your feet are behind the roller pads and your knees are pressed against the seat. Keep your back straight and slowly straighten both your legs together until they have reached full contraction. Hold for a maximum of 6 seconds, or until you can no longer hold the contraction against the weight.

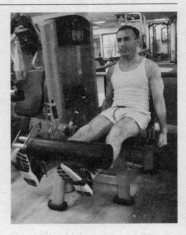

Exercise Two — Leg Curls

Sit on the leg curl machine so that your feet are underneath the roller pads. Slowly curl your lower legs until your heels are close to your buttocks. Keep your back straight and slowly straighten both your legs together until they have reached full contraction. Hold for a maximum of 6 seconds, or until you can no longer hold the contraction against the weight.

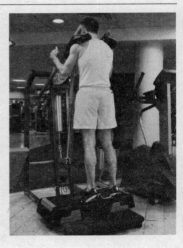

Exercise Three – Standing Calf Raises

Place your shoulders underneath the pads on a standing calf machine. With the balls of your feet firmly placed on the platform, slowly raise up your heels until you are on tiptoes and your calves are in a fully contracted position. Hold for a maximum of 6 seconds, or until you can no longer hold the contraction against the weight.

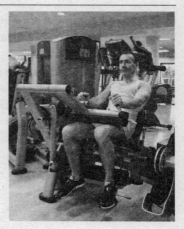

Exercise Four – Lat Pulldowns

Position yourself on the lat pull-down machine. Focusing on the strength of your latissimus dorsi muscles of your back, pull down until your back is in a fully contracted position. Hold for a maximum of 6 seconds, or until you can no longer hold the contraction against the weight.

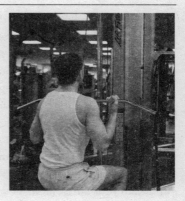

The Live-Long Code

Exercise Five – Shrugs

The safest way to perform this exercise is
on a universal gym machine. Grasp hold of
the barbell and stand up straight with your
back flat, keeping your arms full extended.
Now just using the strength of your trapezius
muscles, shrug your shoulders upwards.
Hold for a maximum of 6 seconds, or until
you can no longer hold the contraction
against the weight.

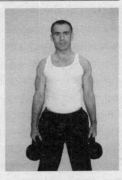

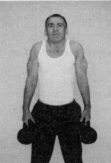

Exercise Six – Cable Crossovers

Grab the cables and draw them
together at waist height. Focus on
using the strength of the pectoral
muscles of your chest. Hold for a
maximum of 6 seconds, or until
you can no longer hold the
contraction against the weight.

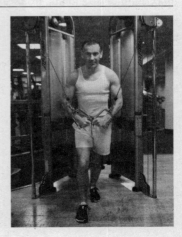

208

Exercise Seven – Lateral Raises

Hold dumbbells at your thighs, and with your back straight smoothly lift the weights up to the sides with your elbows locked and holding at a height just above shoulder level. Hold for a maximum of 6 seconds, or until you can no longer hold the contraction against the weight.

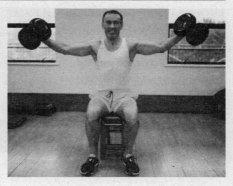

Exercise Eight – Bent Over Laterals

Hold a pair of dumbbells and bend forwards at the waist until your torso is at 90 degrees to your legs. Slowly raise the dumbbells into a position slightly above and behind your shoulders. Hold for a maximum of 6 seconds, or until you can no longer hold the contraction against the weight.

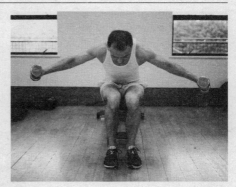

Exercise Nine – Tricep Kickbacks

Holding a dumbbell in your right hand, lean forward on a bench so that your torso and legs are at a 90-degree angle. Contract your triceps behind you so that your arms are fully locked. Hold for a maximum of 6 seconds, or until you can no longer hold the contraction against the weight.

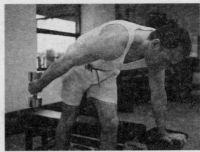

Exercise Ten – Crunches

Lie face up on a floor with your hands behind your head or holding a weight on your chest. Keep your chin on your chest and lift your feet up on top of a bench. From here curl your trunk upwards towards a sitting position. Hold for a maximum of 6 seconds, or until you can no longer hold the contraction against the weight.

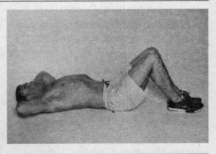

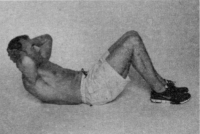

Exercise Eleven – Palms under Close Grip Chin

Place your hands on the chinning bar with an underhand grip. Have your eyes at grip level. Step off slowly and contract your biceps, holding yourself up. Hold for a maximum of 6 seconds, or until you can no longer hold the contraction against the weight.

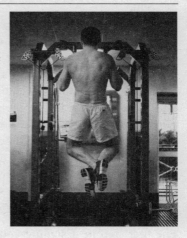

Live-Long Code Cardiovascular Training

Cardiovascular exercise is an important part of the Live-Long Code Exercise Programme. This is aerobic exercise and is one of the great anti-ageing techniques available to us.

The list of the benefits of aerobic exercise is extensive and includes strength gain, fat loss, increased energy, improved breathing and heart function, and an increased sense of well being. In particular, aerobic exercise has been proven to increase HDL (good) cholesterol, lower blood pressure, improve immunity and contribute to protecting the body against a host of illnesses, including stroke, diabetes and osteoporosis.

Research has conclusively proven that cardiovascular exercise increases lifespan. But how much is the right amount? Too little, fairly obviously, has little benefit, but the right amount can have incredibly powerful effects. A study at Harvard University that evaluated 17,000 men aged between 35 and 74 found that as cardiovascular exercise increased, the death rate dropped. Those who expended 2,000 calories a week doing moderate aerobic exercise lowered their overall death rate by 25 to 33 per cent; in particular, their risk of coronary artery disease decreased by an astounding 40 per cent.

On the other hand, studies have also shown that expending 3,500 calories or more a week actually shortened lifespan. So the good news is that a moderate amount of cardiovascular exercise is the key to life extension. It's not fully understood why exceeding this level of training is damaging, but the process of training does increase oxidation, so perhaps if taken to excess this damage outweighs the benefits. Cardiovascular exercise is important for any age group, but it should be tailored to suit the needs of each individual. It is also recommended that you consult your doctor before you start any cardiovascular training programme.

Designing Your Cardiovascular Programme

The first step in designing your cardiovascular programme is to select the type of aerobic exercise you want to take. Scientists have determined that aerobic activities that stimulate breathing by using the large muscle groups in a constant and rhythmical manner are the most beneficial. These include activities such as walking, jogging, running, swimming, cycling and dancing. It is perfectly acceptable to select a number of different aerobic activities to build your cardiovascular programme.

Ideal Duration and Frequency

Approximately 10 to 15 minutes of continuous intensive aerobic activity is the Live-Long Code recommendation for health and longevity. Another way to judge, and the classical measurement of any aerobic exercise, is to look at the number of calories you burn. The Live-Long Code incorporates dedicated cardiovascular exercise three times a week. From an anti-ageing perspective, the frequency of training needed is determined by the calories that you burn over a one-week period. The optimum number of calories (more correctly called kilocalories) to burn during exercise is 2,000 a week. You will burn approximately 800 calories a week weight-training. This means that you should burn 1,200 calories in aerobic exercise – three intensive aerobic sessions at 200 calories per session and 4 walking sessions at 150 calories per session.

Training Intensity

From the point of view of longevity, your goal in cardiovascular training is to exercise at an optimal target heart rate that provides maximum anti-ageing benefits. This is a percentage of your maximum heart rate. Due to the ageing process a young person's maximum heart rate will be different to that of an older person.

The maximum heart rate is easy to calculate and is based on a simple formula: 220 minus your age in years. For example, if you are 40 years old, your maximum is 220 – 40 = 180. This is the maximum heart rate that you should never exceed regardless of the exercise that you are doing; going above this heart rate places undue stress on the heart, and we want the heart to be worked but not over-stressed. In advanced sports and athletics training, over-stressing the heart in this way is quite commonplace as it enables physical improvement and peak performance. It also lengthens the time a long-distance runner can run at faster speeds. But our goal is not to win an athletics competition; it is to extend your life.

From an anti-ageing perspective, around 75 per cent of maximum heart rate is a good level of intensity. Using our previous example, if you are 40 years old, your maximum heart rate would be 180 beats per minute. Seventy five per cent of 180 is 135, so, to exercise at an aerobic level optimal for longevity, your target exercise heart rate should be around 135 beats per minute.

The Aerobic Zone

Our goal is to keep the heart in a healthy condition without over-stressing the cardiac muscles. If you are training at 75 per cent of your maximum heart rate, you will also be increasing your level of endurance. Exercising in this zone will improve your heart function and the number and size of the blood vessels to the heart will increase. You will also see an improvement in overall respiratory function.

The Live-Long Code

Progression

If you consider yourself unfit and haven't trained for quite some time, I recommend that you begin exercising slowly and increase the intensity and length of your cardiovascular training slowly, in increments. Remember that it is only your ultimate goal to reach and maintain 75 per cent of your maximum heart rate; when you are just beginning training your heart rate should be at a level at which you are comfortably able to talk while exercising. In general, aim to increase your intensity by 10 per cent a month. You should feel good after training, not exhausted. Enjoying it rather than torturing yourself will also help to keep up your enthusiasm for training.

If you find that you are exhausted as a result of your exercise programme, then the chances are that you are overdoing it and you need to pull back. Slow down the intensity and shorten the distance.

The Live-Long Code Cardiovascular Workout

It is important to include three phases as part of your exercise programme: the warm-up, the actual exercise workout and the cool down. Each phase has its own particular rationale.

The Warm-Up

The warm-up phase includes the stretching exercises already discussed, which should be performed before strength training exercise. This will loosen your joints and muscles, helping to prevent any undue strain or injury. They also increase your heart rate, which is beneficial in preparing the heart muscles for the workout phase.

The Workout

This phase lasts approximately 10 minutes. To improve cardiovascular fitness and body composition, as well as to lose weight, you will perform continuous cardiovascular exercise at an intensity level of 75 per cent of maximum heart rate. Exceeding this rate is not encouraged as it overstrains the body and increases oxidation, and the resultant free radicals actually cause ageing.

The Cool-Down

This phase lasts just a couple of minutes and enables you to readjust your body back to normal resting level at a gradual pace. Most treadmills and aerobic equipment include a button that automatically sets the equipment for the cool-down phase. This gradual cool-down gives your heart the opportunity to adjust to the decrease in blood flow and helps prevent lightheadedness. This phase also reduces the risk of muscular cramps and stiffness. One of the best cooling-down exercises is simply walking, gradually slowing your pace.

What About Intensity?

When it comes to cardiovascular fitness, the faster you go, the more fuel you use, and the better your heart and your metabolism respond. Although the higher the intensity, the better the aerobic and cardiovascular fitness, exercise should still be tailored to your specific requirements, especially if you are over the age of 40. We know that over-exercising is actually detrimental to your health; therefore you should only perform enough cardiovascular exercise to expend approximately 2,000 calories per week in combination with strength training exercises.

Measuring Progress

In many respects the best tool for judging your improvement should be your mirror rather than your scales. The scales have limitations when it comes to judging results, as, particularly in the early stages of an exercise programme, it is possible to gain muscle as well as lose fat, which will give a misleading reading on the scales.

You can measure your aerobic progress by your ability to increase the duration and intensity of your cardiovascular exercise routine. If you see a slow but steady increase in intensity and duration and find that you can run or cycle at the same speed with less effort, then your cardiac health is improving.

Ultimately, the best measurement of your progress is how good you feel. When you are consistent in your cardiovascular programme, the chances are that you will feel better. If you feel better it's likely that you will look better and generally be in a better frame of mind. This may take a few weeks, but it will come. People around you will notice changes in you after you have been following the programme consistently for a while.

Types of Cardiovascular Exercise

The following table shows the approximate number of calories burned in a 15-minute period when the exercise is performed intensively after strength training exercise. The exact figures will vary depending on a number of factors including the weight and age of the individual as well as the exact intensity of the exercise being performed. The goal is to burn approximately 2,000 calories in total a week, which is what the Live-Long Code Exercise Programme achieves.

	Calories Burned
Walking: 25 mins x 4 days	600
Strength training: 15 mins x 3 days	800
Intensive cardio training: 10 mins x 3 days	600
Total calories burned	2,000

The table can act as a guideline when you're choosing which type of cardio exercise to perform, but ultimately I would recommend that you pick the types of exercise that you enjoy the most and vary them so that you don't get bored; this will make it easier to stick to your routine. I would also recommend that you split your exercise up throughout the day. We will look at some of the more common exercises in turn.

	Calories burned in 15 minutes
Aerobics, high impact	150
Bicycling, fast pace	225
Jogging, 5 mph	150
Rowing, fast pace	200
Running, 8 mph	300
Skipping	215
Stair treadmill	200
Swimming	150
Tai chi/chi kung	80
Tennis	150
Walking, 3.5 mph	80

Walking

Walking is an exercise for everyone and is particularly good for anyone over 40 because of its low impact and safety. Injuries caused by walking are extremely rare, and it is simple and easy to adapt to a busy schedule. A quick walk can burn as many calories as a slow jog. Other benefits of walking include improved cardiovascular health, decreased body fat, a lowered risk of heart disease and a significantly lower risk of cancer.

It makes sense to have the proper footwear. Although there are walking shoes available, some people prefer good running shoes; choose a pair with adequate support and cushioning, especially for the heel, as well as for the forefoot and the arch.

Try to warm up before and stretch and cool down after your walking session. Concentrate on your posture and form; remember to keep your back straight and your abdomen toned and allow your arms to move naturally. If you have a heart monitor, all the better, and your aim should be to walk at a pace that is sufficient to get to and remain at your target heart rate.

Jogging

Jogging is an excellent cardiovascular exercise, and like walking it is popular because of its simplicity and adaptability to a busy schedule. People of all ages can jog, although it is probably more appropriate for those who are in slightly better shape. If you are more than 30 pounds overweight or have knee problems, then it might make sense to begin with walking or another low-impact exercise like swimming instead. When jogging you should focus on your posture; the back should be kept straight and the hands free to move in a natural and relaxed manner. The foot should land heel first, followed by a rolling motion to the front of the foot. Push off for the next step from the ball of your foot. If you are making a lot of noise when you land on the ground, the chances are that you are moving improperly by landing too heavily, which increases the risk of strain and damage to the joints.

Aim to jog at a pace that is sufficient to get to and remain at your target heart rate. This will provide all the benefits of the exercise, without the downside of unnecessary wear and tear on the joints.

Always warm up, stretch and cool down in a jogging session. Begin the session by jogging at low intensity or walking fast. This will stretch your muscles and protect against cramping or injury. After the session, cool down by walking for about 5 minutes, and follow that by stretching the exercised muscles.

Cycling

Cycling's major advantage is that it is a non-weight-bearing exercise and is therefore especially good for people with knee problems or anyone who is overweight, or weaker for any reason. Stationary cycling is common now at most gyms, and cycling outdoors is a perfect activity for those who can use it as a mode of transportation. Cycling is a good exercise for a variety of fitness levels. Once again, posture is important and it is crucial to adjust the height of the seat so that when your leg is at the bottom of the down-stroke it is almost, but not quite, fully extended when your foot is on the pedal. If your seat is too low, you will get tired more easily.

Your speed can vary depending on your fitness level and comfort. Remember to warm up, stretch and cool down. Begin slowly; you can increase your intensity and speed as your fitness improves.

Rowing

This is another excellent cardiovascular exercise and a personal favourite of mine.

Computerised rowing machines are available at most gyms and they offer a safe way of doing cardiovascular exercises. Sit on the seat of the rowing machine and secure your feet. With your body leaning slightly forward, move forward on the roller, bringing your knees close to your chest. Maintain good posture, with your head up and your arms extended straight in front of you. Push back with your legs, straighten your back to an upright position, and pull the rowing handle towards your abdomen. Keep your back straight at all times. A good rate of intensity is approximately 30 rows per minute.

Start your rowing session slowly, giving your muscles time to warm up. After about 2 minutes, or when you have warmed up, you can start to increase your intensity. Remember to cool down towards the end of the session. Rowing offers good variety for your cardiovascular programme as it exercises different parts of the body to most other cardiovascular exercises.

Swimming

Swimming is another excellent non-weight-bearing cardiovascular exercise. It is excellent for those who are overweight or who have injuries. You may wish to take swimming lessons to improve your breathing and swimming skills. Swimming involves using most of the muscles in your body and is therefore a fantastic aerobic exercise. As with all the exercises, warm up, stretch and cool down. Incorporating swimming into your programme along with other cardiovascular exercises provides excellent variety.

Other Exercises

There is a great variety of other cardiovascular exercises to choose from – too many to discuss here! Choose an activity that you enjoy and that has significant cardiovascular benefits. When looking for the exercise that will benefit you the most, ask yourself the following:

- Does the cardiovascular exercise offer a sustained repetitive movement using large muscle groups such as your legs and even better your arms?
- Does it enable you to be continually and intensively active for at least 15 minutes?
- Are you able to maintain an intensity of 75 per cent of your maximum heart rate while performing the exercise?
- Can you continue to pursue these activities for three days a week? (For example, does it depend on weather conditions or access to the gym?)

The key to the Live-Long Code Exercise Programme is to exercise your body in such a way as to promote vigour and reduce stress, as well as increase your longevity. Research now shows that the target aerobic exercise should be of moderate intensity, that is, at a heart rate of approximately 75 per cent of your maximum heart rate, and in sufficient quantity to burn off 2,000 calories per week. Regardless of what exercise you do, these are the key parameters within which you should formulate your exercise programme.

Cardiovascular exercise is an important pillar of the Live-Long Code. By following the guidelines discussed, I believe that you will enjoy yourself at the same time as you are working towards achieving optimum health. The key is putting it into action. Consistent exercise will go a long way towards increasing your longevity. Include cardiovascular exercise in your schedule no matter what it takes. But if you have already taken the time to read this chapter, chances are you have been motivated to understand that this is the right thing to do. So all that is left now is to do it!

Motivation

If you have a day where you feel that you're in need of motivation, why not bear in mind Newton's Law of Motion? This law states that an object at rest will remain at rest, and an object in motion will remain in motion. In other words, it is easier to keep going and make progress when you've started. After the decision has been made, one tiny first step is all that's needed to get the momentum going. On days when you do not feel inclined to exercise, simply make this deal with yourself. Decide to exercise for just 10 minutes instead of the proper 30 – but do it right away. That is all. If after 10 minutes you still don't feel like continuing, then you can stop – but only if you really want to.

This works like a dream. Once you've created momentum, trust me, you will not want to stop after the 10 minutes!

Summary

- Embrace all three elements of the Live-Long Code Exercise Programme: flexibility training, strength training and cardio training. Start off slowly, and as your strength and endurance increases, gradually increase the intensity of your activity.
- Maximise your comfort and safety. Keep warm when you exercise and wear comfortable shoes and clothing. Make sure that you are performing the exercises properly and seek professional guidance. Refer to www.immortalitycode.com for ongoing advice and direction.
- Challenge yourself. Set tough but achievable goals and celebrate every success.
- Enjoy your exercise, and where possible invite friends and family to join in.
- Remember that too much exercise is detrimental to longevity goals, so avoid overtraining.

CHAPTER SEVEN

The Live-Long Code into the Future

Maintaining the most positive psychological framework, avoiding toxic stress, adopting healthy nutrition and optimising your exercise approach all make up a powerful vehicle for hugely positive life changes.

You possess everything you need to implement the Live-Long Code and make it an essential part of your life. You can use it as a catalyst to achieve many of the goals you might have been putting on hold for a long time. At my clinic I have seen thousands of people completely transform their lives. These people often develop a sense of self-worth and life purpose that goes well beyond the obvious physical benefits that accrue from the programme.

Through consistency and determination you will achieve amazing success, going way beyond your expectations. Fantastic goals can become a reality, and the more vividly and intensely you visualise these goals, the sooner they will happen. Realising your full and true potential does require commitment, self-discipline and inner will, but it also requires a sense of enjoyment.

The key to achieving success from this book is to simply put it into practice. It is not just a matter of reading the book, it is also about taking action and implementing the Code. Take responsibility for your health and your longevity and you will find that it is truly liberating and empowering.

The Live-Long Code looks at what you can do for yourself to significantly extend your lifespan. As far-fetched as it may seem, the Live-Long Code might be the tool you need to make you live long enough to see the massive scientific breakthroughs that may just enable people to live forever. Is it as far-fetched as the search for human flight, or putting man on the moon? These are both 'impossible' dreams that have become reality. The longevity scientist Aubrey de Grey has developed his reputation by claiming that some people alive right now could live for 1,000 years or even much longer. According to de Grey, growing old is not an inevitable consequence of the human condition, but rather is the result of accumulated damage at the cellular level that, in time, medical developments will be able to prevent and even reverse. This would mean that lifespan, as well as life in general as we know it, would change completely. Admittedly, most mainstream scientists do not agree with de Grey and most gerontologists refuse to even debate the topic with him, saying that to do so would give credence to his assertions. They avoid discussions about life extension or 'curing' ageing, preferring to focus their attention on keeping older people healthy for longer, a goal referred to in the industry as 'healthspan'.

But to dismiss de Grey as a fantasist is, I believe, a mistake. De Grey is an intelligent, thoughtful and brilliant researcher who has devoted his time and energy to conquering the single biggest medical menace that has consistently faced humanity. Despite his detractors, de Grey has also garnered supporters and gained the respect of some of the world's top scientists.

De Grey has developed a plan that depends on a number of techniques and medical breakthroughs that have yet to happen, such as a cure for cancer. He has called his approach Strategies for Engineered Negligible Senescence (SENS) and it draws on a variety of different scientific and medical disciplines. This strategy has caused somewhat of a stir.

Seven Steps to Immortality

Aubrey de Grey predicts that his seven-step plan will 'cure' ageing, enabling people to live indefinitely. The plan, in theory, would work as follows:

223

1. *The challenge*: Too few cells – cell loss or degeneration.

   The solution: Utilise stem cells (cells that have an ability to renew themselves) to replace lost cells. Or use chemicals that stimulate the continuation of cell division, thus producing new cells.

2. *The challenge*: Chromosomal mutations such as cancer.

   The solution: Genetic therapy can be used to make it impossible for cancer cells to reproduce. Stem cell therapy can be used to avoid side effects.

3. *The challenge*: Mitochondrial mutations.

   The solution: Mitochondria are known as the cell's power plants, and they hold separate genes that are prone to developing mutations that can cause harmful diseases. To prevent such problems, de Grey proposes copying the critical mitochondrial genes and inserting these copies into the cell's nucleus, where they will be better protected.

4. *The challenge*: Too many cells such as fat cells.

   The solution: Possibly inject a chemical to destroy such cells or stimulate the immune system to kill them.

5. *The challenge*: Proteins stiffening outside the cell.

   The solution: Proteins that are outside cells help to support tissues, making ligaments strong and arteries elastic. Chemical reactions occur throughout life and cause those proteins to link up, making them rigid and leading to high blood pressure. Specific chemicals could be used to break these cross-links and enable the proteins to move more freely and easily again. One of these chemicals, ALT-711, is currently undergoing clinical trails.

6. *The challenge*: 'Junk' outside the cell.

   The solution: Plaques can accumulate outside the cell, which can lead to diseases such as Alzheimer's. A vaccine that stimulates the immune system to indefinitely postpone the accumulation of such waste material is currently under development at Elan Pharmacuticals.

7. *The challenge*: 'Junk' inside the cell.

   The solution: As cells age, molecules can change in ways that make them stop working. Those chemical modifications can create structures that cannot be broken down, which consequently accumulate in cells and eventually overwhelm them. Extra enzymes from bacteria could be given to cells to degrade the unwanted material.

While these are the seven challenges of ageing, de Grey is not certain that these proposed solutions will fix the problems. Rather, he is convinced that if we resolve these seven challenges, we will have defeated ageing as we know it.

Dr Anthony Atala, a surgeon and researcher from Wake Forest Institute for Regenerative Medicine, clearly sees merit in de Grey's work and has himself made a remarkable breakthrough. Dr Atala has shown how he and his colleagues are capable of growing new human tissue and organs — bladders, kidneys, blood vessels and cartilage – in the laboratory using the patient's own cells. This means that a few healthy cells could be taken from a cancer-stricken bladder and then used to grow a new healthy bladder, which could theoretically then be transplanted with a very low chance of rejection. In 1999 Dr Atala's team successfully transplanted a lab-grown bladder into a dog, and this procedure has now also proven effective in humans. Dr Atala can take a small section of the patient's bladder, about the size of a thumbnail, and within weeks can bioengineer these cells into a bladder, which can then be grafted back into the patient.

Another researcher making huge breakthroughs in medical science is Dr Woo Suk Hwang of South Korea. Dr Hwang and his colleagues at Seoul National University were the first to successfully clone a dog, a feat that had eluded scientists for years, as dogs are considered to be one of the most difficult animals to clone due to their unique and complex reproductive system. Dr Hwang has since then cloned human embryos and created 11 stem cell lines that are genetically matched to11 patients. This is a medial breakthrough that many scientists believed would not be achieved for decades, and yet it has happened already.

The ability of stem cells to rejuvenate has drawn much attention recently. There is hope that this form of therapy will be used in the near future to treat Parkinson's disease, multiple sclerosis, Type 1 diabetes and Alzheimer's disease, as well as many other conditions effectively. There is also the possibility that stem cells could be used to help people paralysed with spinal cord injuries to regain mobility. At the University of California, paralysed rats have been treated with stem cell therapy and have regained the ability walk.

The hope of stem cell research is that it could be used to create entirely new and complex organs. If this were achieved, someone suffering from heart disease could have a new heart – grown from their own cells. This would make real the possibility of having replaceable body parts, with organs tailored specifically to the patient's body with consequently minimal chances of rejection. There are layers of complexity involved in achieving this but if medical scientists were to meet this challenge it would bring us a number of steps forward along the road towards practical immortality.

Yet another scientist, Cynthia Kenyon, a professor of biochemistry and biophysics at the University of California, has also made some important discoveries. By altering a gene in a roundworm, she has managed to increase its lifespan from two weeks to 20 weeks. This may or may not have implications for humans, but just consider – if we could achieve the equivalent, human lifespan would be increased to almost 800 years.

Aubrey de Grey believes that most medical scientists in the world are in a 'pro-ageing trance'. That is, they believe that ageing and death are inevitable and therefore it is best not to waste time thinking about it. He likens this to the great minds who for centuries ignored the possibility of human flight. However, in 1903 the Wright brothers became the first to sustain a controlled and powered heavier-than-air (or non-balloon) human flight. The impossible had suddenly become reality. What if something similar could happen with ageing? What if ageing *was* preventable and death was no longer a foregone conclusion?

De Grey isn't the first person to propose such an idea, and history is littered with prophets of eternal life. However, what makes de Grey different is that he is a bona fide and devoted scholar. Although he does have many detractors in the science community, a recent $20,000 reward offered to any gerontologist who could prove that his radical theories about life extension were flawed did not produce a winner. For de Grey this was seen as a great victory, and he believes that medical science can no longer ignore him.

One of de Grey's staunchest supporters is Graham Pawelec, Professor of Immunology at the University of Tübingen in Germany. He puts great stock in de Grey's 'escape velocity' theory; the idea that within the next 20 years science will have advanced sufficiently to enable people to live for between 150 and 200 years, and that by the time that these people turn 200, science will have progressed to the point that they will be able to live to 500. According to Pawelec, it isn't that the battle against ageing will soon be over but rather that there will be enough steady progress for us all to potentially live forever.

'In 10 years, we will have proof that we can cure these seven things and therefore beat ageing,' Pawelec says. 'All of my mainstream colleagues will be up there saying Aubrey was right. And then the general public will believe it.'

However, even at de Grey's own conferences there is no shortage of doubters. David Finkelstein from the National Institute on Ageing believes that to claim that by solving these seven problems we will live to be 1,000 is hyperbole. Finkelstein also has little respect for de Grey's own research contributions, although he does admire his ability to act as a provocateur and to ruffle feathers.

The big question is whether de Grey's assertions will prove to be true or not. Dr Gregory Fahy, a biologist and vice-president and chief scientific officer of a biomedical research company, was sceptical at first but now he is largely won over. 'If you think you're right, you have to stand up and say what you believe even if people think you're nuts,' he says. 'Now, if they prove you're nuts, you have to shut up. But that hasn't happened yet.'

So will de Grey be proved correct and we will all live to be 1,000? For me it is hard to imagine that we are so close to conquering death; some major medical breakthroughs are needed, and by their very nature, these breakthroughs are very hard to predict. I do believe that it is inevitable that average lifespan will continue to increase, but whether this will mean that we all live to be 1,000 or a 'mere' 150, I cannot say. What I can say, however, is that by implementing the Live-Long Code you give yourself a better chance of being around to take advantage of any great medical break-throughs. Over time and as new research emerges, the details of the Live-Long Code itself may change, but I believe that the core concepts will remain the same. By maintaining the correct mental approach to healthy ageing, having optimal nutrition, supple-ment and exercise regimes and reducing your exposure to harmful toxins, you will be taking many of the steps currently available to us to extend your healthy lifespan.

When I myself got sick in 1998, as part of my recovery I resolved to make myself healthier each year. Now, in 2009, I have reached the momentous fortieth year of my life, and despite being very athletic in my youth I can confidently say that I am now at the fittest and healthiest that I have ever been. It is going to be a challenge to continue to improve beyond this point and yet that is precisely what I am going to endeavour to do.

The purpose of this book is to help you develop good health and consequently prolong and improve your life. As we age, most of us become increasingly aware of our own mortality. For some this awareness might come with the first appearance of a wrinkle or grey hair; for others it will occur with the loss of somebody close to them. Perhaps you might even find yourself in the situation of being told you have a life-challenging illness. For me, all of the above reminders of my own mortality have occurred. The truth is that we all have obstacles and challenges to deal with in life. There may well be some things that are completely outside your control, but regarding your health, you can take control of many of the important areas. Stem cell and genetic research offers huge poten-tial for dramatic life extension, probably sooner than you might have thought. In the meantime there is much that you can do to take charge of your mind, your body and your health.

In this, my fortieth year, and with serious ill health in my past, I have made a firm commitment to continue my own quest for immortality. If I fall short I'll settle for a prolonged, healthy and happy life. I've watched my children grow so fast and I want to be around for them for as long as I can be. I have lived the guidelines within this book and seen my health continue to improve and my body regain a youthful vigour so fast and so substantially that it shocked me and everyone who knows me.

My mental well being has also significantly improved. Like many people in recent times, the collapsing economy has presented its own special challenges for me. I experienced a degree of stress beyond anything I had encountered before. Being tested in such a way required a positive reaction and I embraced the Live-Long Code in its entirety. Thankfully, seizing a healthier lifestyle is something you can do without spending a lot of money. Indeed, in the long term it will prove to be much more cost-effective than frequent encounters with ill health. I have offered you the best advice that I can find and I hope I have presented it in a way that will help you to make significant changes and improvements to your own life.

Who knows how far along the road to immortality we are? You are in the driving seat, with this book as your map. Please be part of the Live-Long Code community and share with me your own success stories by e-mailing dermot@immortalitycode.com. I wish you a long and healthy life, but most of all I hope that you enjoy the journey.

Until we meet, I would like to send you a blessing:

> *May love and laughter light your days,*
> *and warm your heart and home.*
> *May good and faithful friends be yours,*
> *wherever you may roam.*
> *May peace and plenty bless your world*
> *with joy that long endures.*
> *May all life's passing seasons*
> *bring the best to you and yours!*

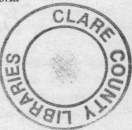

Four months after   Before

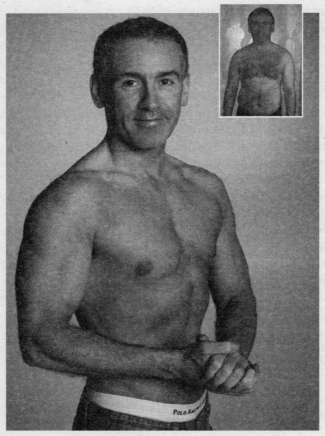

Spend the day with
Dermot O'Connor

If you would like a personal consultation with Dermot O'Connor, or to take part in one of his workshops in the UK or Ireland, visit www.immortalitycode.com or telephone +44 (0) 871 218 0300 (UK) or +353 0 1 667 2222 (Ireland).

Bibliography

Bailie-Hamilton, Paula, *Stop the 21st Century Killing You* (Vermillion, 2005)

Campbell, Phil, *Ready Set, Go!: Synergy Fitness for Time-Crunched Adults* (Pristine Publishers, 2004)

Campbell, T. Colin and Campbell II, Thoma M., *The China Study* (Benbella Book, 2000)

Coleman, Daniel and the Dalai Lama, *Destructive Emotions* (Bantam Books, 2004)

Cordain, Loren, *The Paleo Diet: Lose Weight and get Healthy by Eating the Food you were Designed to Eat* (John Wiley & Sons, 2002)

De Grey, Aubrey, *Ending Aging: The Rejuvenation Breakthroughs That Could Reverse Human Aging in Our Lifetime* (St Martin's Griffin, reprint 2008)

Fichera, Salvatore, *Stop Aging Start Training: Look and Feel Twenty Years Younger* (Basic Health Publications, 2008)

Fitzgerald, Patricia, *The Detox Solution: the Missing Link to Radiant Health, Abundant Energy, Ideal Weight and Peace of Mind* (Ebrandedbooks.com, 2001)

Hicks, Angela and Hicks, John, *Healing Your Emotions: Discover Your Five Element Type and Change Your Life* (HarperCollins, 1999)

Hitchcox, Lee, *Long Life Now* (Nelson Books, 1996)

Johnson, Jerry Alan, *Chinese Medical Qigong Therapy* (Redwing Book Company, 2000)

Kurzweil, Ray, Grossman, Terry, *Fantastic Voyage: Live Long Enough to Live For Ever* (Rodale, 2005)

Kyriazis, Marios, *Carnosine and Other Elixirs of Youth: The Miraculous Anti-Aging Supplement* (Watkins, 2003)

Larre, Claude and de la Vallée, Elizabeth, *Chinese Medicine from the*

Classics: the Seven Emotions – Psychology and Health in Ancient China (China Books, 1996)

Levy, Thoma E., *Optimal Nutrition for Optimal Health* (Keats Publishing, 2001)

Martin, Paul, *The Sickening Mind: Brain, Behaviour, Immunity and Disease* (Flamingo, 1998)

Lipman, Frank, *Total Renewal: 7 Key Steps to Resilience, Vitality, and Long Term Health* (Penguin, 2005)

Little, John, *Max Contraction Training: The Scientifically Proven Program for Building Muscle Mass in Minimum Time* (McGraw Hill, 2003)

Little, John and McGuff, Doug, *Body by Science: A Research Based Program to Get the Results You Want in 12 Minutes a Week* (McGraw Hill, 2009)

McKenna, Paul, *Change Your Life in 7 Days* (harmony, 2005)

Murphy, Joseph, *The Power of Your Subconscious Mind* (Bantam, New York, 2001)

Pert, Candace B., *Molecules of Emotion: Why You Feel the Way You Do* (Pocket Books, 1999)

Pitchford, Paul, *Healing with Whole Foods: Asian Traditions and Modern Nutrition* (North Atlantic Books, 2002)

Plant, Jane and Tidey, Gill, *The Plant Programme: Eating for Better Health* (Virgin Books, 2005)

Rossi, Ernest Lawrence, *The Psychology of Mind-Body Healing: New Concepts of Therapeutic Hypnosis* (W.W. Norton & Co., 1994)

Somer, Elizabeth, *Age-Proof Your Body: Your Complete Guide to Looking and Feeling Younger* (McGraw Hill, 2006)

Snowdon, David, *Aging With Grace: The Nun Study and the Science of Old Age: How We Can All Live Longer, Healthier and More Vital Lives* (Harper Collins, 2001)

Walford, Roy L., and Walford, Lisa, *The Anti-Aging Plan: Strategies and Recipes for Extending Your Healthy Years* (For Walls Eight Windows, 1994)

Weeks, David and James, Jamie, *Secrets of the Superyoung* (Villard Books, 1998)

Wilcox, Bradley, Wilcox, Craig and Suzuki, Makoto, *The Okinawa Way: How to Improve Your Health and Longevity Dramatically* (Mermaid Books, 2001)